THE NATIONAL TRUST
BOOK OF
HEALTHY EATING

COOKERY BOOKS PUBLISHED BY THE NATIONAL TRUST

The Book of National Trust Recipes

The National Trust Book of Fish Cookery

THE NATIONAL TRUST
BOOK OF
HEALTHY EATING

Sarah Edington

Illustrations by Soun Vannithone

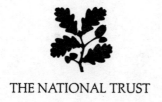

THE NATIONAL TRUST

For my family and friends
who ate with appreciation and
whose comments were always constructive

First published in Great Britain in 1990 by
The National Trust
36 Queen Anne's Gate
London SW1H 9AS

British Library Cataloguing in Publication Data

Edington, Sarah
The National Trust book of healthy eating.
1. Health food dishes – Recipes
I. Title   II. National Trust
641.5'637

ISBN 0–7078–0105–2

Designed by Gail Engert

Phototypeset in Monotype Lasercomp Palatino 853

Printed and typeset in England by
Butler & Tanner Ltd, Frome, Somerset

Contents

Acknowledgements

My thanks to all the cooks who gave me these recipes:

Maggie Black

Sophie Blunn

Kaye Bussell

Joe Coombs

June Cox

Clare Cremin

Ann Denford

Maureen Dodsworth

Joan Easterbrook

Sybil Gill

Jonathon Glinos

Harry Hawkins

Lesley Hunt

Gillian Hunter

Paul Jennings

Rita Jones

Chris Keating

David Lee

Sharon Luke

Annabel Marsh

Shelagh Matthews

Margaret Milner

Joanne Montgomery

Carol O'Mahony

Theresa Owens

Rosemary Pannell

Anne Parkin

Gillian Pickering

Chris Pritchard

Shirley Santos

Joe Shaw

Joan Simmons

Julie Simmons

Di Smallman

Maureen Smith

Sheila Stockdale

Karin Stone

Valerie Stone

Katherine Taylor

Melanie Thomas

Diana Tilbury

Barbara Twiss

Hilary Watkins

Brenda Watson

The Trust would like to thank Alice Ferguson for her assistance, and Victor Gollancz Ltd for their kind permission to quote from *Mistress of Charlecote*.

We Eat to Live – or Live to Eat?

In the Western world in the 1990s, few of us eat simply to live. Food *is* necessary for life, but it is also a vital part of social activities. A dish made with carefully chosen ingredients, cooked with attention and eaten by the cook with family or friends, is a pleasure for all the participants.

Our earliest ancestors did, however, eat to live. Avebury, now protected by the National Trust, is a prehistoric settlement, probably constructed in about 2000 BC. Excavation and research have posed more questions about why the stones of Avebury are there and what they were used for, than provided answers about the lives of the men and women who dwelt there. We do know, however, that their diet was basically vegetarian, using cultivated crops, nuts and berries, with occasional meals of meat or fish provided by the hunter in the family. This was probably the original pattern of eating for *Homo sapiens*, still followed in parts of the Third World.

But what is a healthy diet? Nutritionists, cooks, doctors, dentists, farmers and politicians have debated this knotty problem for years. Every pressure group has its fanatics: we have been told that red meat is a killer; bran is best; yoghurt will help digestion; polyunsaturated fats help to reduce cholesterol; that highly processed foods can be toxic; that all products except those organically grown can damage you. In the end, the messages are so frightening, it's a wonder we eat at all. There's also a danger of overkill.

This book contains recipes using a variety of vegetables and fruit, milk products, nuts, flours, pulses, spices and herbs, but no meat or fish. It is intended for anyone who likes to eat a non-meat meal as part of their diet, as all their diet, or as a positive contribution to their well-being. Every recipe tastes good – some recipes do use white sugar, butter, alcohol and cream, but they also use fresh vegetables and fruit loaded with vitamins, bran, brown rice, wholewheat flour and yoghurt.

All National Trust restaurants offer a vegetarian dish at lunch time and specialise in cakes and puddings using fresh produce and no additives, such as colouring and chemical flavour-enhancers. For this book, I visited twenty-one properties, all providing interesting, varied menus.

Some of the soups are substantial enough to make a meal in themselves: Leek and Potato Broth from Wallington; Minestrone from Quarry Bank, Styal. Others are subtle and sophisticated, such as Golden Cider Soup from Montacute, with its lovely colour and delicate aroma. Try Ossum Salad from Buckland Abbey with its interesting ingredients and delightful story behind the odd name. I have included half-a-dozen pâtés, some served hot with a piquant sauce as a main course, some perfect as an hors-d'oeuvre or for a light lunch with toast or crusty bread.

Many Trust restaurants are lucky enough to be able to use fresh herbs from their own kitchen gardens, while traditional ingredients – leeks in Northumberland, carrots in Derbyshire, Lancashire cheese in Styal – are a feature in many recipes. I have selected hearty gratins, hot pots and bakes as well as sophisticated dishes such as Spinach and Pinenut Jalousie from Charlecote, or Mushroom and Broad Bean Gougère from Cliveden, which are spectacular enough for any special occasion. I hope the collection of vegetable tarts will inspire any cook stuck for ideas. How about a taste of Italy with a Tomato and Basil Tart using olive oil pastry, from Claremont, or a tart from Montacute with a cheese pastry and a filling of eggs, onions, breadcrumbs and clotted cream, delicately flavoured with bay leaves?

I couldn't visit National Trust restaurants without sampling some of the puddings and cakes for which they are justly famous, but mindful of my quest for healthy eating, I have restricted the selection to fruit- or vegetable-based recipes. Vegetable-based may sound rather odd, but you will find an interesting carrot pudding from Claremont, inspired by an Indian sweetmeat recipe, and no less than five different carrot cakes. Also included are tarts and cakes using locally produced cider and apples, a sugar-free teabread, a scone recipe, and a damp, delectable poppy seed cake.

Since these are mostly family recipes, quantities are also family size and will serve four to six people according to appetite. Where cakes are concerned, I have given a tin size. Some of the soups and salads were difficult to reduce to one-meal quantities and you may well find that they will feed another set of hungry mouths at another meal on the next day! Eggs are all standard size 3 unless otherwise indicated. If no sugar variety is given, use caster sugar. I have given cooking times and temperatures but find from personal experience that these do vary from oven to oven so do regard them more as an indication than an order. Where cakes and sponge puddings are concerned, for instance, the best test is to plunge a stainless-steel skewer into the centre of the cake or pudding – if this comes out clean, the cake or pudding is cooked. Most cakes should be taken out of their tins and cooled on a wire tray after cooking, and stored only after they are cold. Similarly, all biscuits should be cooled on a wire tray and put in a tin only after they are cold. When re-heating dishes, they should be heated until they are bubbling and too hot to eat.

A preoccupation with health is not just a twentieth-century obsession. Interspersed with the recipes and descriptions of the properties you will find fascinating glimpses of our ancestors' attempts to stay healthy and also some of their remedies, simples and concoctions. Some of these look quite palatable, some are totally disgusting, some we still use today; the quest for a healthy, active, enjoyable, long life still goes on.

Conversions

The following approximate conversions are used in this book

$\frac{1}{2}$oz	12g	1 teaspoon		5ml
1oz	25g	1 dessertspoon		10ml
2oz	50g	1 tablespoon		15ml
3oz	75g	1 fluid oz		30ml
4oz	125g	4 fluid oz		100ml
5oz	150g	5 fluid oz		125ml
6oz	175g	8 fluid oz		225ml
7oz	200g	10 fluid oz		300ml
8oz	225g	12 fluid oz		360ml
12oz	350g	15 fluid oz		450ml
1lb	450g			
1$\frac{1}{2}$lb	675g	$\frac{1}{4}$ pint		150ml
2lb	900g	$\frac{1}{2}$ pint		250ml
		1 pint		500ml
$\frac{1}{4}$in	6mm	1$\frac{1}{2}$ pints		750ml
$\frac{1}{2}$in	1.25cm	1$\frac{3}{4}$ pints		1 litre
$\frac{3}{4}$in	2cm	2 pints		1.25 litres
1in	2.5cm			
1$\frac{1}{2}$in	4cm	Gas mark		
2in	5cm	1	275°F	140°C
6in	15cm	2	300°F	150°C
7in	18cm	3	325°F	160°C
8in	20cm	4	350°F	180°C
9in	23cm	5	375°F	190°C
10in	25cm	6	400°F	200°C
12in	30.5cm	7	425°F	220°C
		8	450°F	230°C

American Equivalents

Dry Measures

1 US cup = 50g = 2oz of: breadcrumbs; fresh cake crumbs

1 US cup = 75g = 3oz of: rolled oats

1 US cup = 90g = $3\frac{1}{2}$oz of: desiccated coconut; ground almonds

1 US cup = 100g = 4oz of: suet; grated hard cheese; walnut pieces; drinking chocolate; icing sugar; cocoa; flaked almonds; pasta; frozen peas

1 US cup = 125g = 5oz of: white flour; self-raising flour; currants; muesli; chopped dates; ground roasted almonds

1 US cup = 150g = $5\frac{1}{2}$oz of: wholemeal flour; raisins; cornflour

1 US cup = 175g = 6oz of: apricots; mixed peel; sultanas

1 US cup = 200g = 7oz of: caster sugar; soft brown sugar; demerara sugar; glacé cherries; lentils; long grain and brown rice; flaked and drained tuna fish

1 US cup = 225g = $\frac{1}{2}$lb of: cream cheese; cottage cheese

1 US cup = 300g = 11oz of: mincemeat; marmalade

1 US cup = 350g = 12oz of: syrup; treacle; jam

Liquid Measures

$\frac{1}{4}$ US cup = 60ml = 2 fluid oz
1 US cup = 240ml = 8 fluid oz
2 US cups (1 US pint) = 480ml = 16 fluid oz

Butter, Lard and Margarine Measures

$\frac{1}{4}$ stick = 25g = 2 level tablespoons = 1oz
1 stick ($\frac{1}{2}$ US cup) = 100g = 8 level tablespoons = 4oz

Information very kindly provided by the Good Housekeeping Institution

RECIPES FROM NATIONAL TRUST PROPERTIES

BERRINGTON HALL

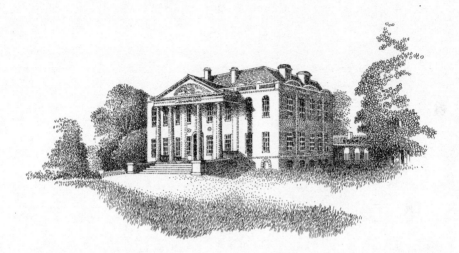

HEREFORDSHIRE is one of England's most beautiful, unspoilt and uncrowded counties: Berrington Hall, an unpretentiously elegant house, lies in rolling hills north of Leominster. The site of the house is wonderful, which is not surprising as it was chosen and later landscaped with the help of Lancelot 'Capability' Brown.

Designed by Henry Holland in 1778, the house is encased in dark red local stone which gives the exterior a slightly austere air, but the interiors provide a complete contrast. The principal rooms have wonderfully delicate ceilings, in particular the Drawing Room, where plaster seahorses and cherubs cavort amongst flowers and leaves, all painted in pastels which have faded to subtly satisfactory blues and lavenders. There is an exquisite Boudoir, a fine Library with interesting ceiling paintings of eminent literary Englishmen, a workman-like Business Room, a handsome, airy staircase hall, and a cool, marble entrance hall.

On the walls hang portraits of those associated with Berrington, amongst them Thomas Harley, Lord Mayor of London in 1767 who built it, and his daughter Anne, who inherited the house and married George, son of Admiral Rodney. In the Dining Room are four huge dramatic pictures of sea battles in which the Admiral triumphed. During this century the house was owned by the Cawley family which is remembered by portraits, photographs, mementos and toys.

The house was designed and built without one lavatory or bathroom: chamberpots had to be kept behind the shutters, and hip baths were filled with water carried by servants. Their world is entered across the courtyard on the east side of the house, where there is a Victorian laundry with huge drying racks and mangles, a pretty tiled dairy and the Servants' Hall, a large light room with a great dresser and black-leaded range. This is now the restaurant where you can eat Herefordshire Cider Cake and Berrington Pies served by waitresses at blue-and-white check-clothed tables. On the walls are old photographs, menus and a huge ox's head with the following inscription:

> This ox with six wether sheep and a quantity of bread and cider was given to the poor of the Berrington Estates on the arrival of Lord Rodney with his Bride at Berrington – September 12, 1850.

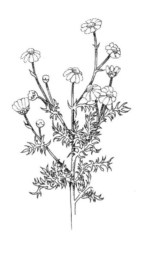

CELERY AND STILTON SOUP

1 medium head of celery, chopped	6 oz (175 g) Stilton cheese
1 medium onion, chopped	3 teaspoons (15 ml) cornflour
2 oz (50 g) butter	$\frac{3}{4}$ pint (400 ml) milk
1 pint (500 ml) vegetable stock	celery leaves, chopped
salt and pepper	

Place the chopped celery and onion in a saucepan and sauté gently in the butter until soft, with a lid on the pan. Pour in the vegetable stock and season with salt and pepper. Bring to the boil and simmer for 20 minutes. Liquidise in a food processor or blender and return to the pan with the crumbled or grated Stilton. In cup or small bowl cream the cornflour with a little cold milk and add to the soup with the balance of the milk. Reheat gently, but do not boil, and check the seasoning. Garnish the soup with a few chopped celery leaves.

Celery and Stilton are both strong flavours; cooked this way the soup enhances both.

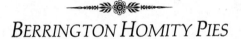

TOMATO, ONION AND GINGER SOUP

1 large onion, chopped
2 tablespoons (30 ml) sunflower oil
1 in (2.5 cm) fresh root ginger, finely
    chopped, or pinch of ground ginger
1½ pt (750 ml) vegetable stock

14 oz (400 g) tin tomatoes
1 dessertspoon (10 ml) tomato purée
fresh herbs of your choice
salt and pepper

In a large saucepan sauté the chopped onion in the sunflower oil together with the ginger until soft and transparent. Add the balance of the ingredients and bring to the boil. Simmer for around 20 minutes, then liquidise in a food processor. Before serving, reheat and adjust the seasoning if necessary.

If you wish, this soup can be thickened with a little cornflour. Do try to obtain fresh ginger as it gives this soup a fresh and unusual tang.

BERRINGTON HOMITY PIES

10 oz (300 g) wholemeal pastry (recipe
    on p. 25)

Filling

12 oz (350 g) potatoes
1 lb (450 g) onions
3 tablespoons (45 ml) vegetable oil
1 oz (25 g) butter
1 tablespoon (15 ml) parsley, chopped

4 oz (125 g) Cheddar cheese, grated
2 cloves garlic, crushed
1 tablespoon (15 ml) milk
salt and pepper to taste

Preheat oven: 425°F, 220°C; gas mark 7.

Roll out the pastry and line six 4 in (10 cm) individual tins — Yorkshire pudding tins are ideal. Boil or steam the potatoes until tender. Chop the onions, sauté in the oil until soft but not coloured. Then combine the potatoes and onions, add butter, parsley, half the cheese, garlic and milk and salt and pepper to taste. Cool, then use to fill the cases. Sprinkle with the remaining cheese and bake in the oven for 20 minutes, until golden.

This Cranks-inspired recipe is a great favourite at Berrington.

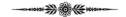

WHOLEWHEAT PANCAKES WITH RATATOUILLE OR MUSHROOM FILLING

Pancake Batter

2 oz (50 g) plain wholewheat flour
pinch of salt
2 eggs

1 tablespoon (15 ml) oil
$\frac{1}{4}$ pt (150 ml) milk
oil for frying

Ratatouille Filling

1 onion, coarsely chopped
2 cloves of garlic, crushed
1 small aubergine, diced into chunks
2 courgettes, sliced
4 oz (125 g) mushrooms, sliced

4 tablespoons (60 ml) olive oil
14 oz (400 g) tin tomatoes
1 teaspoon (5 ml) mixed herbs
salt and freshly ground black pepper

Mushroom Filling

3 oz (75 g) butter
1 oz (25 g) plain flour
$\frac{1}{2}$ pt (250 ml) milk

8 oz (225 g) mushrooms, chopped
salt and pepper
fresh herbs

Make the batter by placing all the ingredients into a food processor and blending for a few seconds until smooth. If you do not have a food processor, put the flour and salt into a bowl and gradually beat in the eggs. Continue beating while adding the oil and milk until a smooth consistency is reached. Brush a small frying pan with oil and make the pancakes in the usual way. Stack them on a plate and keep warm while you prepare the filling.

Ratatouille Filling

Use the ratatouille recipe from Montacute (p. 98)

Mushroom Filling

Make a white sauce by melting half the butter, then stirring in and cooking the flour for a few seconds. Gradually add the milk, stirring all the time, until the mixture comes to the boil and a thick sauce is made. Sauté the mushrooms in the remaining butter and add to the white sauce with seasoning and fresh herbs.

Place a good tablespoon of filling on each pancake and roll up. Serve immediately or reheat in the oven brushed with a little melted butter.

MACARONI CHEESE AND TOMATO BAKE

8 oz (225 g) dried macaroni
1 medium onion, chopped
1 tablespoon (15 ml) oil
14 oz (400 g) tin tomatoes, drained
1 dessertspoon (10 ml) tomato purée
dried mixed herbs or fresh basil

salt and pepper
3 oz (75 g) butter
2 oz (50 g) plain flour
1 teaspoon (5 ml) mustard
$\frac{3}{4}$ pt (400 ml) milk
8 oz (225 g) cheese, grated

Preheat oven: 400°F, 200°C; gas mark 6.

Boil the macaroni in the usual way according to the instructions on the packet and drain well.

Fry the chopped onion gently in a little oil and add the drained tomatoes, tomato purée and plenty of herbs. Cook together for a few minutes, breaking the tomatoes with a wooden spoon and adding salt and pepper to taste.

Make a cheese sauce: melt the butter in a saucepan, stir in the flour with a teaspoon of mustard and cook for a minute before pouring in the milk. Stirring all the time, bring to the boil and add 6 oz (175 g) of the grated cheese.

Stir the tomatoes into the cooked macaroni and spoon into individual baking dishes. Cover each portion with the cheese sauce and sprinkle some grated cheese on top. Bake in the oven for 20 minutes or until golden brown.

HEREFORDSHIRE CIDER CAKE

8 oz (225 g) caster sugar
8 oz (225 g) butter
1 lb (450 g) self-raising flour
1 teaspoon (5 ml) ground ginger

$\frac{1}{2}$ teaspoon (2.5 ml) ground nutmeg
4 eggs
$\frac{1}{2}$ pt (250 ml) cider

Preheat oven: 325°F, 160°C; gas mark 3.

Grease and line a 9 in (23 cm) cake tin. Cream together the sugar and butter until light and fluffy. Sieve the flour and spices into the mixture and gently fold in with a wooden spoon. In a separate bowl whisk together the eggs and cider, then stir them into the cake mixture. Spoon into the cake tin and bake in the centre of the oven for approximately 45 minutes. Turn out on to a wire tray to cool before glazing with glacé icing made with cider (4–6 oz [125–175 g] icing sugar to 1–2 tablespoons [15–30 ml] cider).

At Berrington this is, of course, made with local Herefordshire cider.

BOX HILL

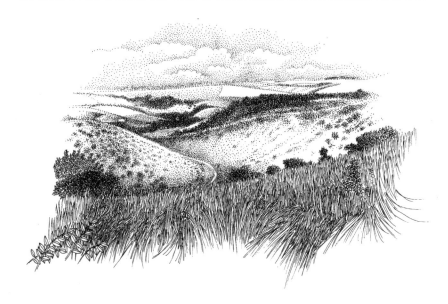

Box Hill is a commanding chalk promontory of woodland and open rolling downland with a steep 400 foot drop to the River Mole on the south and west. One of the best-known summits of the North Downs, it provides on a clear day a vista across the Weald to the tower on Leith Hill (also in the care of the National Trust) and even to Chanctonbury Ring 25 miles to the south and Windsor Castle to the north west. Jane Austen chose the hill as the site of a picnic in *Emma*:

> Emma had never been to Box Hill; she wished to see what every body found so well worth seeing, and she and Mr Weston had agreed to choose some fine morning and drive thither. Two or three more of the chosen only were to be admitted to join them, and it was to be done in a quiet, unpretending elegant way . . .

Like Jane Austen's Emma Woodhouse in 1816, I, too, in 1988 had never been to Box Hill on the edge of the North Downs, though I already knew I would find there fine views, pleasant walks and interesting trees, plants, birds, animals and insects.

In Emma's day, excursions to Box Hill were by carriage, but with the coming of the railway in 1860, the fresh air, lovely woods and exceptional views were accessible to everyone and Box Hill became, and still is, a great favourite with Londoners of all ages.

In all seasons, the walker will find chalkland flowers blooming at their feet, delicate cowslips, pyramid and bee orchids, mallow and harebells. In the summer, butterflies with enchanting names flutter amongst the grasses: silverspotted skipper, chalkhill blues and marbled whites. The bird life is wonderful; tiny tits co-exist with woodpeckers, tree creepers, woodpigeons and tawny owls. A flash of blue down by the river is a kingfisher, the shyest of birds. The lucky visitor may also catch a glimpse of the shyest of animals, the roe deer, browsing in the open woodland in the misty early morning or at dusk. Many of these plants and creatures are becoming increasingly rare with the encroachment of building and pollution, making Box Hill an important reserve and a welcome haven for the natural world.

Walking, kite-flying and birdwatching all encourage healthy appetites and high on the hill is the Old Fort Restaurant. It is surprising that the low white building with wooden verandah blends in happily with its beautiful woodland surroundings, since it is a legacy of a ring of forts constructed between 1893 and 1902 for the defence of London. There is a good old-fashioned doorscraper and doormat for muddy shoes, while the white walls, Windsor chairs and polished boards give a comfortable, rustic atmosphere. The food is substantial and imaginative. The restaurant is open for lunch and tea all the year round.

CURRIED PUMPKIN SOUP

2 medium onions, coarsely chopped
2 tablespoons (30 ml) oil
1 tablespoon (15 ml) Madras curry
   paste
2 lb (900 g) pumpkin
1 large potato, diced
2 pt (1.25 l) vegetable stock
5 fl oz (125 ml) sour cream or yoghurt

Lightly fry the onions in the oil for about 5 minutes; do not colour. Add the balance of the ingredients and simmer gently for around 40 minutes or until the vegetables are soft. Purée in a food processor or blender and reheat before serving. Add a swirl of sour cream or yoghurt, which will also help to smooth off the curry flavour if a little hot, and decorate with sprigs of fresh herbs.

If you can find Queensland Blue (Australian) pumpkins, they are the best for soup because they are much drier than most others and will blend better. The soup can be made thicker with the addition of extra potato.

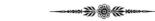

CHEESE AND CELERY SOUP

1 head of celery

1 large carrot

1 large onion

$1\frac{1}{2}$ pt (750 ml) vegetable stock

salt and pepper

6 oz (175 g) Cheddar cheese, grated

Trim the celery and slice, peel and chop the carrot and onion and place in a saucepan with the vegetable stock and seasoning. Bring to the boil, reduce the heat and simmer for about 1 hour, until the vegetables are quite soft. Purée the soup in a blender or food processor. Reheat in the saucepan and add the grated cheddar cheese. Serve with the leaves from the heart of the celery.

The chef recommends that this soup be eaten on a cold day in front of the fire with a glass of port and a fresh wholemeal bread roll!

BOX HILL VEGETABLE PIES

$1\frac{1}{2}$ oz (40 g) butter

1 oz (25 g) plain flour

$\frac{1}{2}$ pt (250 ml) milk

1 teaspoon (5 ml) English mustard

salt and pepper

1 lb (450 g) puff pastry

$\frac{1}{2}$ pt (250 ml) tomato sauce

8–10 oz (225–300 g) mixed cooked

vegetables which can include

potatoes or pulses

parsley, tarragon or coriander (or

mixture)

$\frac{1}{2}$ pt (250 ml) cheese sauce

1 beaten egg

Preheat oven: 425°F, 220°C; gas mark 7

Make a white sauce by melting the butter, then stirring in and cooking the flour for a few seconds. Gradually add the milk, stirring all the time, until the mixture comes to the boil and a thick sauce is made. Add the mustard and season with salt and pepper. Sprinkle in 5 oz (50 g) of the grated cheese and heat gently until it has melted into the mixture.

Roll out the pastry into a large rectangle and divide into 6–8 squares. On one half of each square place a good spoonful of tomato sauce, followed by a spoonful of vegetables on top. Season with salt and pepper, some fresh herbs and cover with cheese sauce. Gently fold over the other half of the pastry and seal the edges well with a little of the beaten egg. Make a couple of small slits in the pastry, brush with the remaining beaten egg and place the pies on a baking sheet. Bake in the oven for 15–20 minutes.

This is a particularly nice way to use any leftover cooked vegetables.

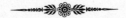

Spinach Tortellini
with Tomato and Basil Sauce

12 oz (350 g) fresh or frozen tortellini

Tomato and Basil Sauce

1 medium onion

2 cloves of garlic

2 tablespoons (30 ml) oil

14 oz (400 g) tin Italian plum tomatoes

3–4 stalks of fresh basil leaves, chopped

Worcestershire sauce

salt and pepper

Cook tortellini as directed on the packet.

To make the sauce, chop the onion and garlic and place in a saucepan with the oil and cook over a medium heat until the onion is soft and transparent. Add the tomatoes, basil leaves, a few drops of Worcestershire sauce and seasoning and cook for around 20 minutes, stirring every now and then to break up the tomatoes until the sauce has thickened. Process lightly in a blender or food processor until the sauce is coarsely chopped and still retains some texture. Pour over and combine with the pasta and serve with a green salad.

Carrot and Walnut Loaf

5 oz (150 g) butter

1 teaspoon (5 ml) vanilla essence

6 oz (175 g) caster sugar

2 tablespoons (30 ml) golden syrup

2 eggs

8 oz (225 g) carrots, grated

6 oz (175 g) raisins or dates

4 oz (125 g) chopped walnuts

10 oz (300 g) self-raising flour

$\frac{1}{2}$ teaspoon (2.5 ml) ground nutmeg

$\frac{1}{2}$ teaspoon (2.5 ml) cinnamon

Preheat oven: 350°F, 180°C, gas mark 4.

Grease and line a 2 lb (900 g) loaf tin with greased paper. Cream together the butter, essence and sugar until light and fluffy. Add the golden syrup and beat in the eggs one at a time until well mixed. The mixture may look curdled at this stage but do not worry. Stir in the carrots, raisins and walnuts and gently fold in the flour and spices. Turn into the loaf tin and bake in the oven for $1\frac{1}{4}$ hours. Leave for 5 minutes before turning out. Serve in buttered slices.

This loaf will keep for about 1 week in a tin or wrapped in foil and will also freeze well.

APRICOT AND ALMOND SHORTCAKE

10 oz (300 g) self-raising flour
5 oz (150 g) butter
4 oz (125 g) caster sugar
1 egg
1 tablespoon (15 ml) lemon juice

1–2 tablespoons milk (optional)
6 oz (175 g) apricot jam
1 egg white, lightly beaten
1 oz (25 g) halved almonds

Preheat oven: 350°F, 180°C; gas mark 4.

Well grease an 8 in (20 cm) flan tin. Sift the flour into a large bowl and rub in the butter to resemble fine breadcrumbs. Stir in the sugar, egg and lemon juice and draw together to make a light, manageable dough; use a little milk as well if necessary. Place in a polythene bag in the fridge to rest for approximately 30 minutes. Divide dough in half and roll out one half between two sheets of cling film; this makes it much easier to handle. Press it evenly into the base of the tin and slightly draw it up the sides. Heat the jam and spread it over the dough, leaving a small clear margin around the edge. Roll out the remaining dough and place over the jam, pressing the edges firmly together. Brush with the lightly beaten egg white and decorate with the halved almonds. Bake for approximately 30 minutes, or until golden and firm and leave to cool for 10 minutes before turning out.

No fresh fruit or vegetables in this, but it is economical, crisp and good warm or cold. This shortcake will keep for around 3 days and is also suitable for freezing.

FRESH FRUIT KEBABS

Strawberries
Chunks of apple, pears or bananas
    dipped first in lemon juice
Cherries (stoned)

Pineapple
Melon
Mangoes

Thread 3 or 4 different fruits on a 6 in (15 cm) stick. Arrange them in a circle on a large platter decorated with, say, vine leaves. Place in the centre a small bowl of Greek yoghurt mixed with soft brown sugar to taste. Guests then help themselves and use the yoghurt and sugar as a dip.

This can be particularly colourful and perfect for a crowd.

BROWNSEA ISLAND

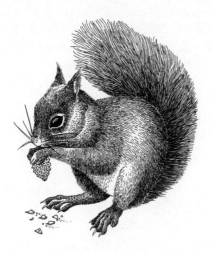

Just half an hour from Poole Town, or ten minutes from Sandbanks across Poole Harbour's busy waterway, is a small island where time is governed by the natural cycle of the seasons, where birds, animals and plants flourish in their natural surroundings, safe from pollution and predators. It is a world away from the stress of life on the mainland.

Brownsea Island is only 500 acres, but it contains an astonishing variety of habitats and inhabitants: seabirds love the marsh and mudflats of the lagoon; delicate oystercatchers, plaintive curlews, godwits, redshanks and greenshanks and sixty avocets feed and nest there in the winter. In the spring and autumn, they are joined by thousands of migratory visitors. In the summer graceful terns breed on specially made gravel islands. Colourful shelduck, cormorants and gulls roost here all year round.

Freshwater marshes and wet woodland support twenty-four different types of dragonflies, diving beetles and waterboatmen, tasty meals for warblers, tits, moorhens and finches. Wildflowers with lovely names — marsh orchids, ragged robin, lady's-smock — fast disappearing from our often destructively farmed countryside, can all be found on the marsh edge. Sixty types of tree grow here, sheltering butterflies, fungi, rabbits, mice and shy Sika deer. At night, tawny owls hunt, and seven varieties of bat have been recorded.

The pines on the western side provide food for Brownsea's most celebrated resident, the red squirrel. Almost extinct on the mainland, overwhelmed by its pushy American grey cousin, it lives here happily on pine cones and seeds. Despite a reputation for shyness, the red squirrel is bold enough to investigate litter bins.

23

Brownsea has had a mixed history. In Roman times, the tiny community provided pottery for the army of occupation in Britain. Ravaged and pillaged by the Vikings, Brownsea then became a home for smugglers. In strong contrast, the island was to be the site of the first scout camp when Robert Baden-Powell was encouraged by the owner to hold an experimental camp for twenty boys of differing background in 1907. The island's last private owner, Mrs Bonham-Christie, was a recluse whose desire for solitude and love of nature ensured that Brownsea retained its unspoilt character in a time of unprecedented change.

The Cafe Villano is one of a cluster of cottages built originally by the excisemen in their fight against smugglers. Here you can find a good soup or a tasty baked potato to satisfy an appetite sharpened by walking nature trails, watching birds or just wandering in this enchanting place.

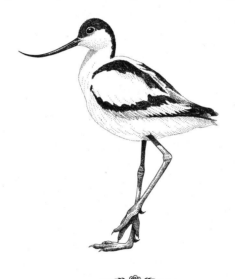

PARSNIP AND ONION SOUP

1 lb (450 g) parsnips, coarsely chopped
1 medium onion, coarsely chopped
1 teaspoon (5 ml) dried basil
3 oz (75 g) butter
4 tablespoons (60 ml) flour

1½ pt (750 ml) vegetable stock
sprigs of fresh coriander
salt and pepper
¼ pt (150 ml) single cream

In a large saucepan sauté the onion, chopped parsnips and dried basil with the butter for five or ten minutes. Stir in the flour; cook briefly, and gradually add the stock together with the fresh coriander. Simmer gently until tender and season to taste with salt and pepper. Allow to cool a little, then liquidise in a blender or food processor. Reheat to serve and at the last minute add the cream and a few leaves of coriander for decoration.

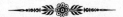

LENTIL AND ONION SOUP WITH LEMON

1 large onion, chopped
3 oz (75 g) butter
1 teaspoon (2.5 ml) dried tarragon
3 pt (1.75 litres) vegetable stock
8 oz (225 g) red lentils

3 tablespoons (45 ml) lemon juice
salt and pepper
$\frac{1}{4}$ pt (150 ml) single cream (optional)
lemon slices

Chop the onion and sauté in a large saucepan with the butter and tarragon for five minutes. Pour in the stock, add the lentils and bring to the boil. Simmer for around 20 minutes or until the lentils are cooked. Season to taste with the lemon juice and salt and pepper. Pour into bowls, swirl in some cream and decorate with a lemon slice.

The thickness of this soup can be varied by using more or less water. It is not necessary to liquidise it unless you require a really smooth texture.

This will make a generous quantity of soup.

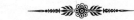

CELERY, APPLE AND MUSHROOM QUICHE

Pastry

6 oz (175 g) plain wholemeal flour
2 oz (50 g) plain white flour
pinch of salt

2 oz (50 g) butter
2 oz (50 g) vegetarian lard
2 tablespoons (30 ml) cold water

Filling

4 oz (125 g) Cheddar cheese, grated
2 oz (50 g) butter
3 sticks of celery, sliced
5 oz (150 g) button mushrooms

2 apples, one green and one red
mixed herbs
6 eggs
salt and pepper

Preheat oven: 425°F, 220°C; gas mark 7

Grease a 9 in (23 cm) loose-bottomed flan tin. In a large bowl mix together the flours and salt. Cut the fats into pieces, then using your fingers, rub the fats until the mixture resembles fine breadcrumbs. Add the water and gently gather the pastry together into a ball. Turn out on to a floured board and knead lightly, then roll out to the required size. Line the tin with the pastry and prick the base with a fork. Cook in the oven until set for approximately 15 minutes.

Lower oven heat to: 350°F, 180°C; gas mark 4.

For the filling, sprinkle the cheddar cheese over the base of the flan.

Soften in butter the sliced celery and mushrooms separately, and slice or coarsely chop the apples, leaving the skins on. Arrange the fruit and vegetables in lines on top of the cheese, lightly cover with herbs, season with salt and pepper, and pour in carefully the beaten eggs. Place the flan in a moderate oven and bake for 30 minutes.

The selection of fruit and vegetables makes good contrasting textures, and if you lay them out carefully it will look particularly pretty.

----※ ❁ ※----

BAKED POTATO TOPPINGS

The quantities of the toppings below are for two jacket potatoes.

Spicy Beans

1 large tin baked beans
1 clove of garlic, crushed

$\frac{1}{2}$ teaspoon (2.5 ml) chilli
    powder/cayenne
1 teaspoon (5 ml) cumin

Heat all the ingredients together in a saucepan and pour over the baked potatoes.

This recipe is very easy but it makes a hearty meal for the hungry.

Mushrooms and Courgettes in a Garlic Cream Sauce

2 oz (50 g) butter
3 cloves of garlic, crushed
1 heaped teaspoon (6 ml) dried basil
8 oz (225 g) button mushrooms
2 courgettes, sliced

1 tablespoon (15 ml) flour
$\frac{3}{4}$ pt (400 ml) milk
mustard and cress, and tomato slices to
    garnish

Melt the butter in a saucepan and cook the garlic and dried basil gently to release the flavour. Add the whole button mushrooms and courgettes and cook for a minute or two before stirring in the flour. Pour in the milk and bring to the boil, stirring frequently, until you have a thick creamy sauce. Serve over the jacket potatoes. This recipe can look a little grey so garnish with a lettuce leaf, chopped mustard and cress and a slice of tomato.

Braised Celery and Mandarins

2 oz (50 g) butter
1 dessertspoon (10 ml) fresh or dried
  tarragon
3 cloves of garlic, crushed
5 sticks of celery, sliced

scant $\frac{1}{4}$ pt (150 ml) water
small can mandarins, drained
salt and pepper
mustard and cress, lettuce or tomato to
  garnish

Melt the butter in a saucepan and gently cook the tarragon and garlic for a minute or two to bring out the flavour. Add the sliced celery and braise over a low heat for 5 minutes. Pour in the water, cover tightly with a lid and simmer for 10 minutes or until tender. Spoon in the mandarins, season to taste with salt and pepper and heat through. Serve out with a slotted spoon and garnish with lettuce, mustard and cress or tomato.

Stilton and Pineapple

2 oz (50 g) butter
2 tablespoons (30 ml) flour
$\frac{3}{4}$ pt (400 ml) vegetable stock
4 oz (100 g) crumbled Stilton

sprig of fresh coriander
salt and pepper
small can pineapple chunks

Make a roux by melting the butter in a saucepan, stirring in the flour and cooking over a gentle heat for 2–3 minutes. Add the vegetable stock gradually, stirring all the time, and bring the sauce to the boil. Sprinkle in the crumbled Stilton, coriander and 2 tablespoons pineapple juice. Season to taste with salt and pepper, then heat gently but do not boil. Just before serving, add the pineapple chunks.

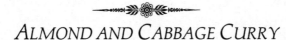

ALMOND AND CABBAGE CURRY

4 oz (125 g) butter
2 cloves of garlic, crushed
4 oz (125 g) split almonds (not flaked)
$\frac{1}{4}$ large white cabbage, cut into $\frac{1}{2}$ in
  (1.25 cm) strips

1 tablespoon (15 ml) Madras curry
  paste
$\frac{1}{2}$ teaspoon (2.5 ml) dried basil
1 tablespoon (15 ml) flour
1 pt (500 ml) vegetable stock
1 tablespoon (15 ml) peanut butter

Melt the butter in a large saucepan and sauté the garlic for a few seconds before adding the split almonds and the strips of cabbage. Cook for a minute, then stir in the curry paste and dried basil. When this is all incorporated into the mixture, sprinkle in the flour and continue to cook for around 30 seconds. Gradually pour in the vegetable stock and bring to the boil. Stir in the peanut butter and simmer for half an hour.

Serve with wild/brown rice and garnish with a few sprigs of watercress, accompanied with a side salad and chutneys of your choice.

Dumb-bell at Knole

For many years a dumb-bell stood in the attic gallery above the Billiard Room at Knole in Kent. The apparatus resembled a double-ended windlass: from its weighted roller a rope passed down through the floor to the room below, to be pulled rhythmically by the user, causing the roller to rotate, first to wind, then unwind the rope. With the considerable effort required to do this, the user would thus guarantee himself – and it must have been a himself – plenty of exercise.

The dumb-bell's age is a mystery. Reference to their use appear in eighteenth-century writings, such as Joseph Addison: 'I exercise myself an hour every morning upon a Dumb Bell that is placed in a corner of my room ... The landlady and her daughters are so well acquainted with my exercise that they never come into my room to disturb me while I am ringing.' It has been suggested that the device was installed at Knole by Elizabeth I's cousin, Thomas Sackville, 1st Earl of Dorset, some time after taking over the house in 1603. It is now in the kitchen lobby, and not accessible to visitors. However, the rope may be seen hanging from the ceiling in the Billiard Room.

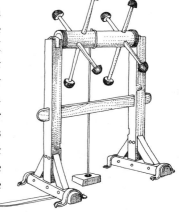

BUCKLAND ABBEY

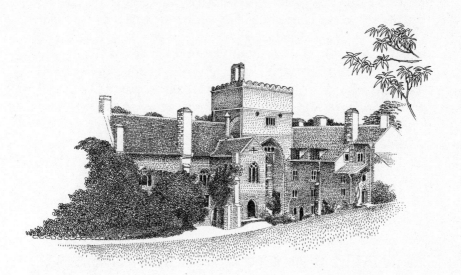

Deep in the lush green valleys that separate Devon from Cornwall lies Buckland Abbey. It is a wonderfully peaceful place now, but it has not always been so; during its long history, the fortunes of its owners have been caught up in some of the more turbulent events of medieval and Tudor England.

In the Middle Ages, Buckland was a great Cistercian monastery – a self-sufficient community founded in 1278 by Amicia, Countess of Devon and endowed with over 20,000 acres of land which were farmed by the monks. Their success can be measured by the size of the Great Barn, bigger than the Abbey Church itself, which was built to store produce from the farms. Eight centuries on, it is still an awesome experience to stand in this huge building.

Dissolved by Henry VIII in 1539, the Abbey was bought by Sir Richard Grenville, whose son Roger lived there until he was drowned with 500 of his men in the ill-fated *Mary Rose*. His heir, the Richard Grenville of *Revenge* fame, completed and converted the Abbey buildings into a fine country house. The splendid Great Hall, has, high on its walls, spectacular plasterwork showing vivid allegorical scenes, including a resting knight, his shield and skull hung above him on the 'tree of life'.

There was a disastrous fire here in 1938 but luckily the plasterwork survived, as did the beautiful oak panelling in the Drake Chamber. Buckland Abbey's most famous owner was Sir Francis Drake, Queen Elizabeth's favourite buccaneer and explorer, and, of course, the man who played a leading role in the English fleet that defeated the Spanish Armada, once he had finished his game of bowls on Plymouth Hoe. Distant relations of Drake continued to live at Buckland until the twentieth century, a Georgian Sir Francis introducing an elegant staircase and fitting out a handsome dining-room. There are interesting exhibitions to visit on Drake, his contemporaries and his career as well as the Abbey itself through the ages.

Stroll back past the Great Barn, the sweet-smelling herb garden and the Linhay, to the long building on your right opposite the Ox Shed, which was the Guesthouse. Now it houses a beautiful restaurant – a long low room with white-washed walls and two great fireplaces at either end, full of flowers. Fennel, sage, thyme, tarragon and other herbs picked fresh from the garden enhance the delicious and unusual recipes you will find here. Try the Spinach and Cream Cheese Pâté or the unusual salads. The hot dishes are substantial and imaginative, and at coffee or tea time, the poppy-seed cake must not be missed.

Sir Francis Drake's sailors were chiefly provisioned on biscuit, salt beef and beer when at sea: 1 lb (450 g) biscuit and 1 gallon (4.5 litres) beer a day, 2 pieces salt beef or $\frac{1}{4}$ stockfish or pieces of saltfish on four days of the week with 4–8 oz (125–225 g) cheese and butter on the other days, supplemented by any fruit, vegetables or fresh meat the captain could procure.

This diet, with its absence of fresh vegetables and fruit, brought on scurvy: 'swollen limbs with haemorrhages under the skin, and foul mouths with swollen, ulcerated and bleeding gums.' Sir Richard Hawkins, who set sail for the South Seas in 1593 and was particularly struck by scurvy among his men, knew of the use of oranges and lemons, but believed the primary cause to be 'the ayre of the land – for the sea is natural for fishe – and the land for men'.

Although seamen on long voyages were particularly prone, peasants in the Middle Ages probably suffered from scurvy too, especially in late winter and spring when their diet contained practically no fresh vegetables and certainly no fruit. By the sixteenth century some drying and pickling of fruit and vegetables were being done in the south of England, but until the end of the sixteenth century even those who never went to sea were in at least a pre-scorbutic condition by the end of the winter.

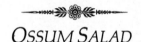

SPINACH PÂTÉ

1 lb (450 g) frozen spinach, defrosted
   and drained well
3 hardboiled eggs
8 oz (225 g) cream cheese

3 tablespoons (45 ml) double cream
1 dessertspoon (10 ml) Worcestershire
   sauce
salt and pepper

Put everything in a food processor and blend until smooth. Check the seasoning and pack into 6 ramekin dishes. Chill before serving. This pâté will keep for several days in the fridge.

An unusual first course, or serve with French/granary bread and a salad as a light meal.

OSSUM SALAD

8 oz (225 g) tinned or cooked red kidney
   beans
3 tablespoons (45 ml) French dressing
1 small onion, finely chopped
4 sticks celery, finely chopped

1 small cauliflower broken into florets
$\frac{1}{2}$ red pepper cut into strips
$\frac{1}{2}$ green pepper cut into strips
$\frac{1}{4}$ pt (150 ml) soured cream or yoghurt
salt and pepper

Heat the beans gently, then pour over them the French dressing while they are still warm. When they have cooled down, add the remaining ingredients and gently mix everything together. Chill and serve.

It is so called because the original writer of the recipe was visiting American friends when this salad was served. Their son declared, 'Gee Mom, this is an ossum salad'. Intrigued by the name the writer enquired for the recipe, to be told the young man had in fact said the salad was AWESOME! It was therefore always named Ossum Salad.

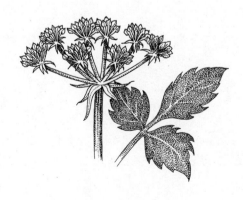

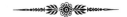

CARROT, RAISIN AND SESAME SEED
SALAD

6 carrots
3 oz (75 g) raisins

1 oz (25 g) sesame seeds
orange and lemon juice dressing

Coarsely grate the carrots and mix in the raisins and sesame seeds. Garnish with lemon twists and pour over an orange or lemon juice dressing. The dressing from Kedleston (p. 88) is delicious with this salad.

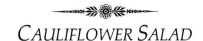

CAULIFLOWER SALAD

1 medium cauliflower cut into florets
3 tablespoons (45 ml) mayonnaise
2 tablespoons (30 ml) double cream

1 tablespoon (15 ml) tomato purée
dash of Worcestershire sauce
salt and pepper

Place cauliflower florets in a bowl. Mix together the balance of the ingredients for a dressing and pour over the florets and garnish with parsley.

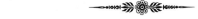

CUCUMBER AND DILL SALAD WITH A
HONEY, LEMON AND LIME DRESSING

1 cucumber
salt and pepper

2 tablespoons (30 ml) fresh dill, chopped
(if fresh not available, use slightly
reduced quantity of dried)

Dressing
1 tablespoon (15 ml) lemon juice
2 tablespoons (30 ml) runny honey

1 tablespoon (15 ml) lime juice (use
another lemon if not available)

Slice the cucumber and season with salt and pepper. Add 1 tablespoon of chopped dill and let it stand for approximately $\frac{3}{4}$ hour in a cool place. Drain off any liquid and pour over the dressing. Garnish with the remaining tablespoonful of dill. You will need to serve this with a slotted spoon.

The sweet and sour combination of this salad is unusual and refreshing.

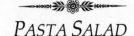

PASTA SALAD

8 oz (225 g) pasta shells
1 bunch of spring onions
$\frac{1}{2}$ green pepper

French dressing
edible flowers such as nasturtiums or
violets

Cook the pasta shells according to instructions in boiling water and drain well. Chop the spring onions and pepper, add them to the pasta and pour over the French dressing. Garnish the salad with flowers.

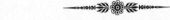

ORANGE AND NUT ROAST
WITH YOGHURT AND ORANGE SAUCE

Orange and Nut Roast

1 oz (25 g) butter
1 medium onion, chopped
2 large eggs (size 1 or 2)
4 oz (125 g) brown bread-crumbs
1 teaspoon (5 ml) mixed herbs
8 oz (225 g) chopped mixed nuts
grated zest of an orange

1 small parsnip, cooked and mashed
juice of an orange made up to $\frac{1}{2}$ pt
    (250 ml) of liquid with vegetable
    stock
1 teaspoon (5 ml) yeast extract
salt and freshly milled pepper

Yoghurt and Orange Sauce

6 fl oz (180 ml) natural yoghurt
2 tablespoons (30 ml) double cream,
    lightly whipped

zest and juice of one orange
2 oz (50 g) onion, finely chopped

Preheat oven: 350°F, 180°C; gas mark 4.

Sauté onion in butter until soft. Leave aside to cool a little. Beat eggs in a bowl large enough to take all the ingredients. Add bread-crumbs, herbs, nuts, orange zest and onion, mix well and add finally the mashed parsnip. Dissolve the yeast extract in the vegetable stock and juice and add to the other ingredients. Taste and season accordingly with salt and pepper.

Prepare a 1 lb (450 g) loaf tin by lining the base and sides with silicon paper. Then turn the mixture into the lined tin and press down well. Cover with foil and cook for 30–40 minutes. Remove foil and cook for a further 10 minutes. Turn out, eat hot or cold with Yoghurt and Orange Sauce, which is made by simply mixing the ingredients together.

Optionally 2 oz (50 g) of grated mature cheddar can be added to the roast mixture.

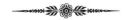

BRAZIL NUT ROAST

1 oz (25 g) butter	1 small cooked swede, mashed
1 medium onion, chopped	$\frac{1}{4}$ pt (150 ml) vegetarian stock
2 large eggs	$\frac{1}{4}$ pt (150 ml) red wine
4 oz (125 g) brown bread-crumbs	1 teaspoon (5 ml) yeast extract
$\frac{1}{2}$ teaspoon (2.5 ml) dried basil	1 tablespoon (5 ml) peanut butter
$\frac{1}{2}$ teaspoon (2.5 ml) dried marjoram	salt and freshly milled pepper
8 oz (225 g) chopped Brazil nuts	

Red Wine Sauce

1 tablespoon (15 ml) oil	$\frac{1}{2}$ pt (250 ml) vegetable stock
1 medium onion, peeled and finely	$\frac{1}{4}$ pt (150 ml) red wine
chopped	salt and freshly milled pepper
1 clove of garlic, crushed	arrowroot or cornflour to thicken
$\frac{1}{2}$ teaspoon (2.5 ml) mixed herbs	

Preheat oven: 350°F, 180°C; gas mark 4.

Sauté onion in butter until soft. Leave aside to cool a little. Beat eggs in a bowl large enough to take all the ingredients. Add bread-crumbs, herbs, nuts and finally the mashed swede and mix well. Dissolve the yeast extract in the wine and stock and add to the other ingredients together with the peanut butter. Season to taste with salt and pepper.

Prepare a 1 lb (450 g) loaf tin by lining base and sides with silicon paper. Then turn the mixture into the lined tin and press down well. Cover with foil and cook for 30–40 minutes. Remove foil and cook for a further 10 minutes. Turn out, serve with Red Wine Sauce or alternatively the Mushroom and Red Wine Sauce from Kedleston (p. 85).

To make the sauce, sauté in the oil the onion and garlic in a small saucepan until soft but not coloured. Add herbs, stock and wine and simmer until liquid is reduced by approximately one third. Season with salt and pepper and thicken to taste with a little arrowroot or cornflour.

This nut roast would make a good vegetarian Christmas dish.

VEGETABLE CROUSTADE

For the Base
2 oz (50 g) almonds

1 oz (25 g) sesame seeds

2 oz (50 g) walnuts

1 oz (25 g) cheese

3 oz (75 g) bread-crumbs

1 teaspoon (5 ml) mixed herbs

salt and pepper

3 tablespoons (45 ml) oil/butter

Topping
3 oz (75 g) cheese, grated

3 oz (75 g) breadcrumbs

1 oz (25 g) sesame seeds

Vegetable Mix
4 oz (125 g) butter

2 medium-sized onions, chopped

1 lb (450 g) vegetables (peppers, celery,
   carrots, cauliflower, leeks,
   courgettes), chopped

salt and pepper

$\frac{1}{2}$ teaspoon (2.5 ml) grated nutmeg

1 tablespoon (15 ml) soy sauce

4 oz (125 g) mushrooms

2 dessertspoons (20 ml) flour

$\frac{1}{2}$-$\frac{3}{4}$ pt (250–400 ml) milk

Preheat oven: 350°F, 180°C; gas mark 4.

Coarsely chop all the nuts and mix with the grated cheese, bread-crumbs and herbs and season with salt and pepper. Mix in the oil to make a soft crumble-type texture. Press into a greased round or deep ovenproof dish and bake for 15 minutes.

To make the vegetable mix, melt butter in a large pan and add the onions. Cook gently for a couple of minutes then add all the chopped vegetables except the courgettes, salt and pepper, grated nutmeg and soy sauce and continue cooking until they are barely tender and still crisp. Add the mushrooms (and courgettes if using), simmer for a further minute, then coat the mixture with flour. Pour in the milk and cook until the sauce thickens (not too runny). Cover the base with the vegetable mixture and cook for 20 minutes. After 10 minutes put on the mixed-together topping ingredients. Serve hot with a salad.

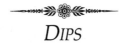

DIPS

With all dips, adjust seasoning as necessary

Blue Cheese Dip

3 oz (75 g) Danish Blue/Stilton
2 oz (50 g) cream cheese
1 oz (25 g) Cheddar cheese
1 tablespoon (15 ml) mayonnaise

1 tablespoon (15 ml) single cream
1 tablespoon (15 ml) lemon juice
pinch of salt

Blend all ingredients to a smooth cream and serve with chunks of French bread or raw vegetables.

Avocado Dip

1 medium avocado
2 tablespoons (30 ml) single cream
dash of Worcestershire sauce

pinch of cayenne pepper
1 tablespoon (15 ml) grated onion
1 tablespoon (15 ml) lemon juice

Mash the avocados with the cream to a smooth purée. Add remaining ingredients and mix together. Serve with raw vegetables or cheese biscuits.

3 oz (75 g) of cream cheese may also be blended with the other ingredients. To stop any discolouration, store with the avocado stone submerged in the dip.

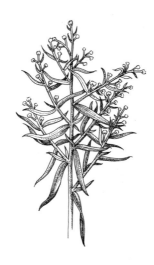

Garlic Dip

2 cloves of garlic, crushed
2 tablespoons (30 ml) mayonnaise

2 tablespoons (30 ml) single cream
salt and pepper

Mix all the ingredients together and serve with raw vegetables.

Tomato Dip

8 oz (225 g) tomatoes
1 small onion
1 clove of garlic or garlic paste
1 tablespoon (15 ml) dried marjoram

a little tomato purée
pinch of sugar
salt and pepper

Put the tomatoes in hot water, then in cold and peel off the skins. Chop up
the flesh, finely chop the onion and combine all the ingredients in a liquidiser
or blender and process until you have a thick smooth sauce.

Serve with long stick bread and raw vegetables.

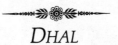

DHAL

8 oz (225 g) lentils (red split lentils,
    continental green lentils, green or
    yellow split peas can be used)
1 large onion, chopped
2 tablespoons (30 ml) vegetable oil
1 level teaspoon (4 ml) mustard seed
1 teaspoon (5 ml) crushed or ground
    cumin

1 teaspoon (5 ml) crushed or ground
    coriander
1 teaspoon (5 ml) turmeric
salt and black pepper
2 tablespoons (30 ml) lemon juice, or
    mix lemon and lime juice together

Soak lentils for 1 hour, drain and add approximately 1 pt (500 ml) of cold
water. Bring to the boil and simmer gently for 20–30 minutes until the
water is absorbed and the mixture is thick and mushy. Sauté the onion
lightly in oil. Add all the spices, except lemon/lime juice, and stir into the
onion for a minute or two over a low heat. Take off the heat and stir in the
lemon/lime juice with the lentils.

Fresh root ginger, grated and added with lemon/lime juice, adds extra
umph!

OATMEAL SODA BREAD

1 lb (450 g) wholemeal flour
4 oz (125 g) fine oatmeal
1½ teaspoons (7.5 ml) cream of tartar
1 teaspoon (5 ml) bicarbonate of soda

1 oz (25 g) butter
¾ pt (400 ml) milk/water mix
1 teaspoon (5 ml) salt

Preheat oven: 350°F, 180°C; gas mark 4.

Mix together the flour, oatmeal, cream of tartar and bicarbonate of soda. Using your fingers, rub in the butter to resemble fine breadcrumbs. Add the milk/water and mix to a soft dough. Turn out the mixture on to a lightly floured surface and knead slightly into a loaf shape or slightly flattened round ball. If you wish, the surface can be deeply scored with a knife in portions. Place on a greased baking sheet and bake in the oven for 30–35 minutes.

Easy and quick to make, delicious to eat straight from the oven or cold with a salad, pasta, croustade or nut roast. Soda bread does not keep well and should be eaten in 1 or 2 days.

POPPY-SEED CAKE

4 oz (125 g) blue poppy-seeds
8 fl oz (225 ml) milk
8 oz (225 g) butter or margarine
8 oz (225 g) light raw cane sugar

3 eggs separated
8 oz (225 g) self-raising wholemeal
    flour

Preheat oven: 350°F, 180°C; gas mark 4.

Grease and line an 8 in (20 cm) cake tin. Bring the poppy-seeds to the boil in the milk, turn off the heat and leave them to soak for 25 minutes in the covered pan.

Cream the butter and sugar together until light and fluffy. Add the egg yolks, one at a time, and beat thoroughly. Fold the flour gently into the creamed mixture and stir in the seeds and milk. Whisk the egg whites until stiff and carefully incorporate into the mixture. Spoon it into the prepared tin and bake for 1–1¼ hours or until the centre is firm and the cake has stopped 'singing'. Let it stand for 10 minutes, then turn out to cool.

CALKE ABBEY

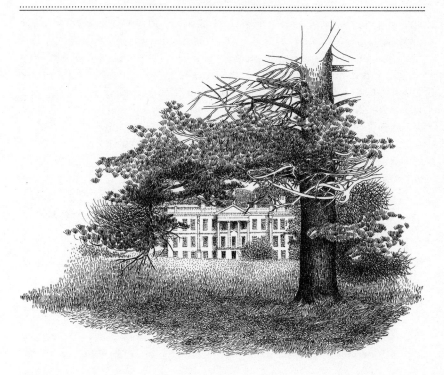

CALKE ABBEY lies deep and secluded in 750 acres of parkland, rich in ancient trees, landscaped by the reclusive Harpur Crewe family, to remain a private, secret place. The house is a Baroque mansion built by Sir John Harpur at the beginning of the eighteenth century. Externally very little alteration has been made since 1841, while inside Calke is the house 'where time has stood still'. Since 1886, when Sir Vauncey Harpur Crewe, the last great collector in a family of passionate collectors, inherited the house practically nothing has changed. Calke presents a unique glimpse of life in a late Victorian household.

Henry Harpur-Crewe, Sir Vauncey's grandson, gave Calke to the National Trust in 1985. With the help of grants from the National Heritage Memorial Fund, English Heritage and a successful appeal, the Trust took on the mammoth task of arresting 60 years of neglect of the house, with its furniture, pictures and extraordinary eclectic collections: toys and dolls, children's clothes, carriages, musical instruments, walking sticks, and, above all, natural history specimens. The Harpur Crewes were fascinated by minerals, fossils, shells, birds' eggs, skeletons and butterflies, and Sir Vauncey, in particular, was an enthusiastic taxidermist; anything that could be stuffed can be found at Calke, some birds and animals shot and stuffed by Sir Vauncey.

A brave decision was taken. Damp, decay and structural weaknesses have been treated, but the contents of Calke have been left much as they were found; pictures are still dark, fabrics faded but beautiful, the decoration of the rooms in the muted colours that time has given them. The house is a splendid clutter of possessions: stuffed heads of longhorn cattle adorn the Entrance Hall; case after case of specimens fill the Saloon, still captioned in Sir Vauncey's spidery hand; late Victorian furniture crowds the Drawing Room; faded maps and worn leatherbound books line the walls of the Library. One item, however, blazes forth in all its original bright colours: the State Bed, given to the family by the Royal Family in the 1730s. Amazingly it remained for 250 years in its original wrappings, never put up because there was no room high enough to accommodate it.

Away from the rooms of state, the drab paint and lime-washed walls give a salutary glimpse into the hard world of the nineteenth-century 'below stairs'. The kitchen and sculleries are particularly grim, with their walls painted blue to keep away the flies, and the stern abjuration to servants 'to waste not, want not' inscribed over the fireplace.

Outdoor staff fared somewhat better: the smithy, tackroom, brew-house and bakehouse are all in elegant, eighteenth-century buildings. The byres and cattle sheds, now containing the shop and restaurant, are handsome, functional rooms, carefully converted and furnished with elegant modern furniture, lighting and underfloor heating. The menu is imaginative, using local ingredients and with a particularly positive attitude to healthy eating. I ate a superlative mushroom pâté, followed by a delicious sugar-free cake.

Calke Abbey, Wimpole and Erddig all have examples of the pillar shower. These ingenious portable machines, made in the nineteenth century, consist of a cylindrical tank supported on pipes painted to look like bamboo. The hot water was released from the tank and circulated by being pumped up from the catchment tray. At Erddig, a cartoon by John Doyle hangs next to the shower, demonstrating how it worked.

LENTIL SOUP

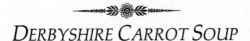

8 oz (225 g) red lentils
2 oz (50 g) onion, finely chopped
2 oz (50 g) carrot, grated
2 pt (1.25 l) vegetable stock

bouquet garni
1 teaspoon (5 ml) tomato purée
salt and pepper

Place the lentils, onion and carrot in a large saucepan and pour in the stock. Add the bouquet garni, tomato purée and bring to the boil. Simmer gently for about 30 minutes until the lentils and vegetables are cooked. Season with salt and pepper and serve with some croutons.

If you are cholesterol conscious this soup is particularly appropriate as it contains no fat.

DERBYSHIRE CARROT SOUP

1 oz (25 g) butter
1 lb (450 g) carrots, grated
1 onion, chopped
1 stick of celery, finely chopped

$1\frac{1}{2}$ pt (750 ml) vegetable stock
2 tablespoons (30 ml) milk
$\frac{1}{2}$ teaspoon (2.5 ml) sugar
salt and pepper

Melt the butter in a large saucepan and stir in the carrots, onion and celery. Cook for 15 minutes, stirring frequently, over a low heat without allowing the vegetables to colour. Pour in the vegetable stock, bring to the boil and simmer for a further 15 minutes. Add the milk and sugar and season to taste with salt and pepper. Serve with a sprinkling of chopped parsley.

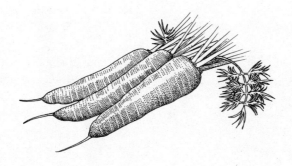

PARSNIP AND TOMATO BAKE

4 oz (125 g) dried pasta shells

2 large parsnips, roughly chopped

2 large leeks, roughly chopped

1½ oz (40 g) butter

1 oz (25 g) plain flour

½ pt (250 ml) milk

1 teaspoon (5 ml) English mustard

salt and pepper

6 oz (175 g) Cheddar cheese, grated

3 large tomatoes, sliced

Preheat oven: 350°F, 180°C; gas mark 4.

Cook the pasta according to the instructions on the packet. Cook the chopped parsnips and leeks in boiling water for 10 minutes. Drain and mix them with the cooked pasta.

Make a white sauce by melting the butter, then stirring in and cooking the flour for a few seconds. Gradually add the milk, stirring all the time, until the mixture comes to the boil and a thick sauce is made. Add the mustard and season with salt and pepper. Sprinkle in 5 oz (150 g) of the grated cheese and heat gently until it has melted into the mixture.

Place half of the vegetable and pasta mixture into an ovenproof casserole dish and layer with slices of tomato covered with half of the sauce. Repeat the layering, then sprinkle the top with the remaining cheese. Bake in the oven for 30 minutes or until the top is golden.

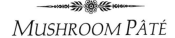

MUSHROOM PÂTÉ

TO FILL FOUR—FIVE RAMEKINS

1 small onion, finely chopped

5 oz (150 g) butter

8 oz (225 g) mushrooms, wiped and
    chopped

1 oz (25 g) fresh white bread-crumbs

4 oz (125 g) full-fat cream cheese

1 teaspoon (5 ml) lemon juice

pinch of nutmeg

salt and freshly ground black pepper

Soften the finely chopped onion in butter and toss the mushrooms for around 30 seconds and cool. Add the bread-crumbs, cheese, lemon juice and seasoning, and turn into the ramekin dishes and chill before serving.

This dish may be served as a first course or as a main meal with salad and crusty bread.

This will keep – even improve – for several days in the fridge.

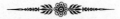

SUGAR-FREE BANANA CAKE

3 oz (75 g) dates
2 fl oz (60 ml) water
8 oz (225 g) ripe (or over-ripe) bananas
1 egg
3 oz (75 g) plain wholemeal flour

1 oz (25 g) bran
1 teaspoon (5 ml) bicarbonate of soda
2 oz (50 g) ground almonds
$\frac{1}{2}$ teaspoon (2.5 ml) vanilla essence
5 fl oz (125 ml) low-fat yoghurt

Preheat oven: 350°F, 180°C; gas mark 4.

Grease and flour a 1 lb (450 g) loaf tin. Place the dates into the water on a low heat until the water is all absorbed. Blend to a smooth paste and then cool. Mash the bananas and whisk the egg and add to the date paste. Lightly fold in the flour, bran, bicarbonate of soda and the ground almonds and gently stir in the vanilla essence and yoghurt. Spoon the mixture into the greased loaf tin and bake for 45 minutes until well risen and just firm. Turn out and cool on a wire rack.

Not only is this a wonderfully healthy recipe but an excellent way of using bananas past their best.

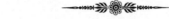

SUGAR-FREE MARMALADE SCONES

5 oz (150 g) plain wholemeal flour
2 oz (50 g) bran
$\frac{1}{2}$ teaspoon (2.5 ml) bicarbonate of soda
1 teaspoon (5 ml) cream of tartar

1 oz (25 g) margarine
2 oz (50 g) sugar-free marmalade
2 teaspoons (10 ml) grated orange rind
2 fl oz (50 ml) skimmed milk

Preheat oven: 450°F, 230°C; gas mark 8.

Mix the flour, bran, bicarbonate of soda and cream of tartar together in a bowl. Rub the margarine into the dry ingredients until the mixture resembles fine bread-crumbs. Gently stir in the marmalade and orange rind and bind with the milk to give a soft dough. Turn out the mixture on to a floured surface and knead lightly before rolling out to approximately $\frac{3}{4}$ in (2 cm) thick. Cut out the scones into rounds using a 2 in (5 cm) cutter and place on a greased baking sheet and bake in the oven for approximately 10 minutes, until brown and well risen. Cool a little on a wire rack.

Try them hot for a special breakfast.

CASTLE DROGO

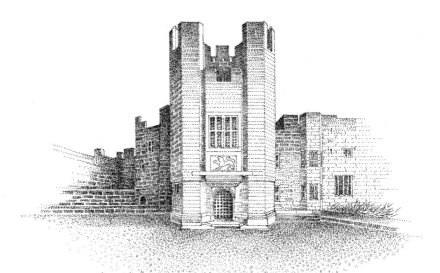

ASTLE DROGO is the last castle built in England, the realisation of a romantic dream for two remarkable men. Julius Drewe founded The Home and Colonial Stores and made a fortune. In 1910, he commissioned Edwin Lutyens to design and build him a great castle. With his son Adrian, he had already chosen the spectacular site. Castle Drogo dominates the Teign Valley in Devon, high up on a spur of Dartmoor, one of the last wildernesses of Britain.

The first sight of this monumental granite pile is breathtaking and yet the building we see now is only one-third of the original design. From the outside Drogo is a true castle, built of huge granite blocks, up to 6 feet thick, cut and worked by hand locally. It has turrets, battlements, arrow slits and a portcullis which works with chains and winches. Above the door is the Drogo motto and the Drogo lion.

Inside the castle the atmosphere is more of a grand country house. The walls are hung with family portraits and tapestries, the furniture is comfortable, the rooms well-proportioned but not forbiddingly large. There are many personal mementoes and reminders of the Drewe family, including a touching family memorial room to Adrian, who was killed in the First World War. The tribute was created by his mother.

Lutyens, like his great predecessor, Robert Adam, concerned himself with detail as well as the grand design. He loved kitchens and he designed everything here from the slate shelves, teak draining boards and the vegetable racks by the back door to the wonderful round table under the vaulted roof, complete with special curved chopping boards. Since this dome provided the servants with their only light, it must have felt like washing up in a cathedral.

The grounds are similarly formal and orderly. Huge, beautifully clipped yews frame lawns where by arrangement visitors can play croquet. Refresh yourself after the game or your tour of the castle in the oak-panelled Servants' Hall and Mr Drewe's study. There are lace tablecloths, a beautiful view over the Teign Valley, and waitresses serving good soups, well-cooked puddings and, of course, superb Devon cream teas!

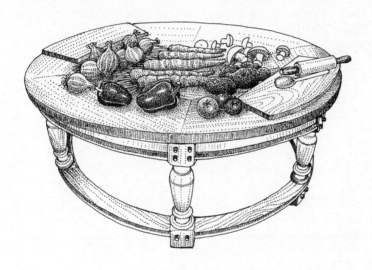

CREAM OF WATERCRESS SOUP

1 medium onion, chopped	*1 pt (500 ml) milk*
2 small potatoes, chopped	*1 pt (500 ml) vegetable stock*
2 oz (50 g) butter	*salt and pepper*
2 bunches of watercress	*8 tablespoons (120 ml) double cream*

Coarsely chop the onion and potatoes and simmer in a large saucepan with the butter until fairly soft but not browned. Pick over the watercress, discarding any yellow leaves, and add to the pan with the milk and vegetable stock. Bring to the boil and simmer for 20 minutes. Cool a little before liquidising. Pour back into the saucepan and season with salt and pepper. Heat gently just before serving, and with each bowlful swirl in a little cream.

The soup is a lovely colour and healthy too – watercress is rich in iron.

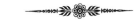

CARROT AND CASHEW NUT SALAD
WITH YOGHURT DRESSING

8 oz (225 g) carrot, coarsely grated   *4 oz (125 g) cashew nuts*
2 oz (50 g) raisins

Dressing
rind and juice of 1 orange   *salt and pepper to taste*
small pot Greek thick yoghurt   *a little crushed coriander (optional)*

Mix salad ingredients together in a bowl. Combine the dressing ingredients and gently stir into the salad. Decorate with chopped coriander or parsley and a twist of orange.

The salad provides a good contrast of creamy, crunchy textures.

MINTY NUT LOAF
WITH A SPICY TOMATO TOPPING

8 oz (225 g) cream cheese   *6 oz (175 g) Brazil nuts, coarsely*
4 oz (125 g) bread-crumbs   *chopped*
8 oz (225 g) chopped mushrooms   *1 egg*
6–8 sprigs mint, finely chopped   *salt and pepper*

Preheat oven: 400°F, 200°C; gas mark 6

Lightly grease a 1 lb loaf tin. Mix all the ingredients together in a large bowl and gently press into the greased tin. Cover with a piece of tin foil and bake in a bain-marie for 45 minutes. Slip a knife around the sides of the tin and turn out on to a warm serving dish.

For the spicy tomato topping use the tomato sauce recipe from Box Hill, Tortellini with Tomato Sauce (page 21), substituting a pinch of chilli powder in place of the basil. Pour a little over the top of the loaf and serve the balance in a sauce boat.

This dish is best served hot with a salad of your choice.

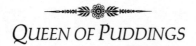

VEGETABLE SCRAMBLE

4 oz (125 g) butter
1 small cauliflower broken into florets
4 sticks of celery, chopped
8 oz (225 g) carrots, sliced
8 oz (225 g) parsnips (if possible), diced
1 lb (450 g) onions, coarsely chopped

12 oz (350 g) tin chopped tomatoes
herbs of your choice (optional)
8 oz (225 g) spinach
12 oz (350 g) tin red kidney beans
   (drained)
salt and pepper

Melt the butter in a large saucepan and add the first five listed vegetables; simmer gently until barely tender. Pour in the tin of tomatoes and continue to cook for a further 5–10 minutes together with any herbs of your choice. In a separate saucepan cook the spinach and when just done add to the other ingredients together with the drained kidney beans. Season with salt and pepper and gently heat through.

This dish can either be served on its own or in a large casserole dish, topped with potato and placed under a grill to brown. Decorate with cress.

QUEEN OF PUDDINGS

1½ pt (750 ml) milk
8 oz (225 g) fresh white bread-crumbs
6 oz (175 g) caster sugar
rind 1 lemon, grated

3 eggs separated
a few fresh strawberries (if available)
3 level tablespoons (13 ml) strawberry
   jam

Preheat oven: 350°F, 180°C; gas mark 4.

Grease generously a 2–2½ pint (1.25–1.5 l) shallow ovenproof dish. In a saucepan heat the milk to boiling point and remove from the heat. Stir in the bread-crumbs, 2 oz (50 g) of the caster sugar and the lemon rind. Leave the mixture to soak for around fifteen minutes. Separate the yolks from the whites of the eggs and beat them into the cooled mixture. Pour it all into the ovenproof dish and bake in a moderate oven for 30 minutes or until the mixture is lightly set. Remove from the oven and cool slightly before placing some fresh strawberries over the top.

In a small saucepan gently melt the jam and pour over the strawberries and filling. Whisk the egg whites until stiff and add the balance of the caster sugar. Continue to whisk until the mixture is stiff and glossy. Spoon or pipe over the top of the pudding and bake for a further 15 minutes until the meringue is lightly browned all over.

With the fresh strawberries this becomes a really superlative pudding.

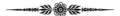

APRICOT BREAD AND BUTTER PUDDING

6 oz (175 g) dried apricots

3 oz (75 g) sultanas

1 lb (450 g) medium-sliced white bread, lightly buttered

grated nutmeg or powdered cinnamon

8 fl oz (225 ml) milk

8 fl oz (225 ml) single cream

6 oz (175 g) caster sugar

vanilla essence

3 eggs, lightly beaten

1–2 teaspoons (5–10 ml) lemon juice

Preheat oven: 350°F, 180°C; gas mark 4.

Soak the apricots in 1 pint (500 ml) water overnight. Generously grease a $2\frac{1}{2}$ pint (1.5 l) soufflé dish. Soak the sultanas in hot water for 10 minutes, drain and mix with 2 oz (50 g) apricots. Remove the crusts from the buttered bread and cut into triangles. With the buttered side up, place in the greased soufflé dish and layer with the sultanas and apricots and a sprinkling of nutmeg or cinnamon. In a saucepan heat together the milk, cream and caster sugar to boiling point. Take off the heat and add a few drops of vanilla essence and the well-beaten egg yolks. Pour the custard over the bread mixture and wait a few minutes for it all to be absorbed. Cover the dish with foil and bake in a bain-marie for 50 minutes or until the pudding is set and firm. Remove from the oven and allow to cool so that it can firm up slightly before turning out on to a serving dish.

To make the sauce, place the remaining apricots and the soaking liquid into a saucepan and simmer for around 15 minutes. Add the balance of the sugar and lemon juice and stir until dissolved. Blend in a liquidiser or food processor and serve separately in a jug.

The apricots add a welcome tang to this traditional pudding.

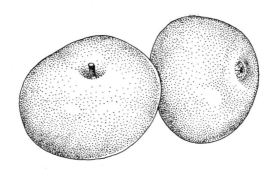

DROGO CARROT CAKE

12 oz (350 g) carrots, grated
3 eggs, lightly beaten
8 oz (225 g) soft dark brown sugar
5 fl oz (125 ml) oil

8 oz (225 g) self-raising flour
$\frac{1}{2}$ teaspoon (2.5 ml) mixed spice
2 oz (50 g) coconut
2 oz (50 g) raisins

Topping for cake

2 tablespoons (30 ml) cream cheese
4 tablespoons (60 ml) icing sugar

lemon juice to flavour
grated lemon or orange rind

Preheat oven: 300°F, 150°C; gas mark 2.

Grease and line a 7 in (18 cm) cake tin. In a large mixing bowl combine together all the ingredients until evenly mixed. Spoon into the cake tin and bake for approximately $1\frac{1}{4}$ hours or until a skewer inserted into the centre comes out clean. Leave to cool in the tin before turning out.

For the topping, beat together the ingredients and spread on top of the cooled cake with a palate knife and decorate with the grated rind.

The coconut, spice and the cream cheese topping give the Castle Drogo Carrot Cake an exotic, tropical flavour.

DEVON CIDER AND APPLE CAKE

1 large cooking apple, peeled and
    chopped
2 oz (50 g) sultanas
scant $\frac{1}{4}$ pt (150 ml) dry cider
4 oz (125 g) butter
4 oz (125 g) soft brown sugar
2 eggs, lightly beaten

8 oz (225 g) wholemeal or plain flour
1 teaspoon (5 ml) baking powder
1 teaspoon (5 ml) allspice
1 teaspoon (5 ml) cinnamon
rind 1 lemon, grated
1 tablespoon (15 ml) demerara sugar
    (optional)

Preheat oven: 350°F, 180°C; gas mark 4.

Grease an 8 in (20 cm) cake tin. Soak the chopped apple and sultanas in the dry cider. In a separate bowl cream together the butter and sugar until light and fluffy. Gradually beat in, little by little, the eggs. Sift together all the dry ingredients and fold into the mixture together with the lemon rind. Add the soaked fruit and cider and gently mix until it is well incorporated. Spoon into the prepared tin, scatter the demerara sugar over the top and bake for 45–60 minutes.

CHARLECOTE PARK

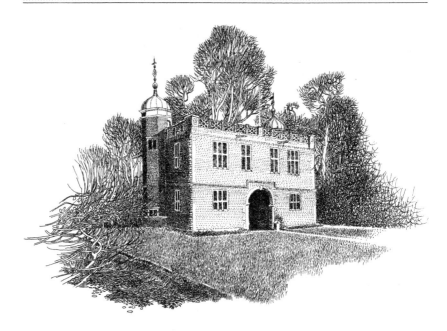

THE Lucy family have lived at Charlecote since the twelfth century, though Sir Thomas Lucy built the present house in 1551. The mellow brick exterior, faded to a delicate rose pink, seems totally Elizabethan but in fact only the Gatehouse is unaltered and authentic – generations of Lucys have made their changes over the succeeding centuries. Legend has it that the youthful William Shakespeare was caught poaching deer in the park. Sir Thomas, the resident magistrate, fined and flogged him in the Great Hall. Fleeing to London to find fame and fortune, Shakespeare immortalised Sir Thomas as the fussy, vainglorious Mr Justice Shallow in *Henry IV Part II* and *The Merry Wives of Windsor*. Deer still roam the park.

By the time George Hammond Lucy inherited in 1823, the estate had become shabby and run down. He married a young Welsh heiress, Mary Elizabeth, and the couple enthusiastically set about restoring the property and redecorating the interior. The result is fascinating; the rooms are rich and to our eyes wonderfully Victorian, but George and Mary Elizabeth saw them as Elizabethan. The Dining Room and the Library, added by George, have heavily ornamented, plastered ceilings, carved oak panelling and richly coloured wallpapers. Some furniture was made specially in Elizabethan style, while seventeenth-century ebony seat furniture – bought because the Lucys thought they had belonged to Elizabeth I – have tapestry seats and backs worked by Mary Elizabeth. The Great Hall, resplendent with family portraits, was also transformed by George Hammond Lucy: its barrel-vaulted ceiling looks like wood but is painted plaster, and so are the stonework walls; even the Elizabethan fireplace is Victorian.

As young bride, mother, widow and grandmother, Mary Elizabeth lived for 60 years in the house and loved every nook and cranny. You can see her Drawing Room decorated in amber silk and furnished with delicate, rather uncomfortable furniture. Her beloved little harp is still sitting in one corner. Above the tackroom in the stables there is an interesting video using excerpts from her diary to bring alive Victorian Charlecote.

When I visited, a local school was learning about spit-roasting in the kitchen. The cool brew-house is full of old machinery and enormous wooden vats. In the stables are the Lucy coaches and the saddles, bridles and coachmen's uniforms.

In the garden, alongside a huge herbaceous border is a delightful thatched summer-house, based on Mary Elizabeth's recollection of her childhood visit to the cottage of the Ladies of Llangollen. She furnished it with child-sized furniture and objects for the amusement of her children. Nearby is the Victorian Orangery now used as the restaurant; feathery green plants, terracotta walls, blue chairs and rush matting give a conservatory atmosphere. Herbs from the garden add a fresh taste to the crisp salads, substaining soups and wholesome hot dishes. Warwickshire apples are famous – light and moist Charlecote Apple Cake is a recipe worthy of them.

TARRAGON AND VEGETABLE SOUP

1 medium onion	1 dessertspoon (10 ml) tomato purée
1 large potato	14 oz (400 g) tin tomatoes
1 medium parsnip	1 dessertspoon (10 ml) tarragon
1 green pepper	(preferably fresh)
1 stick of celery	1 pt (500 ml) vegetable stock
1 large carrot	salt and pepper
2 oz (50 g) butter	$\frac{1}{4}$ pt (150 ml) single cream

Prepare all the vegetables and chop coarsely. Sweat in a large saucepan with the butter until slightly softened. Add the tomato purée, tin of tomatoes, tarragon and enough vegetable stock to cover. Bring to the boil and simmer until all the vegetables are very soft. Process in a liquidiser, return to the pan and reheat. Adjust the seasoning and stir in the single cream before serving.

Tarragon has a delicate yet distinctive flavour – a very underrated herb, well worth growing if you have the chance.

Mary Elizabeth, who married George Hammond Lucy in 1823, wrote an account of her life some sixty years later. This memoir provides a remarkable insight into Victorian life. There are references to accidents and illnesses: in 1883, for instance, Mary Elizabeth recorded a terrible fall downstairs at Charlecote, badly hurting her back. She doctored herself with 'lots of leeches, many poultices, and other disagreeable remedies'.

Her visit to a dentist in 1871 is a telling reminder of how lucky we are with modern methods: 'he put me in his horrid dentist chair and looked into my mouth and at first said all was right, but then began tapping like a woodpecker at every separate tooth, declared that he had found one double tooth that was going – or might go – and before I could get out of his clutches he gag'd me and set to work, positively cutting away half of it, and filling it up with gold which he knocked in with a small hammer till I thought he would hammer my brains out. He thumped and thumped for half an hour, when he was quite exhausted; and then his assistant hammered for another three quarters of an hour, and another young dentist came to look on, and exclaimed "beautiful"! I was frantic, and when at last I did get out of the chair and looked in the glass and saw a nice white tooth (at least half of it) turned into gold, my rage knew no bounds. Yet I had to pay the wretch three guineas.'

GRAPE, MUSHROOM AND PEANUT SALAD

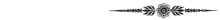

4 oz (125 g) mushrooms, sliced
2 oz (50 g) dry roasted peanuts
8 oz (225 g) black grapes, halved and
 de-seeded

thin coating of French dressing
parsley, finely chopped to decorate

Combine the first three ingredients, pour over the French dressing and gently turn the salad with a wooden spoon. Decorate with the parsley and serve.

This salad is unusual, nourishing and tasty.

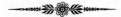

PINENUT AND SPINACH JALOUSIE

$1\frac{1}{2}$ lb (675 g) puff pastry

Stuffing

1 beaten egg (use only half and save
    balance to glaze the jalousie)
3 oz (75 g) fresh brown bread-crumbs
juice and rind of half a lemon

pinch of oregano
pinch of sage
fresh parsley, chopped

Filling

1 small onion, chopped
2 oz (50 g) pinenuts
2 oz (50 g) hazelnuts, chopped

2 oz (50 g) white bread-crumbs
1 beaten egg
pinch of nutmeg

Spinach Mixture

8 oz (225 g) spinach, cooked and well
    drained
4 oz (125 g) Cambazola cheese (or other
    soft, blue cheese)

pinch of nutmeg
freshly ground pepper

Preheat oven: 425°F, 220°C; gas mark 7.

Combine the ingredients of the stuffing and the spinach mixture in two separate bowls. For the filling, fry the onion and mix with the other ingredients. Roll out the pastry into two large rectangles and place one on a greased baking sheet. Leaving a margin round the edge, spread with first the stuffing, then the filling and lastly the spinach mixture. Brush the edge with a little beaten egg and place the second rectangle on top, sealing the edges well. Make horizontal cuts in the top pastry from one side to the other, $1\frac{1}{2}$ in (3.75 cm) apart. Brush with the remaining beaten egg and bake for 30–45 minutes until golden brown.

    Rich and impressive – the green filling surrounded by golden pastry looks lovely and tastes even better!

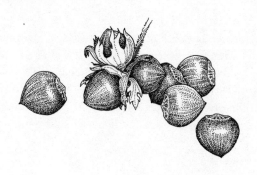

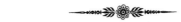

BROCCOLI AND PASTA BAKE

SERVES EIGHT

8 oz (225 g) dry pasta shells	12 peppercorns
8 oz (225 g) broccoli florets	3 oz (75 g) butter
3 pt (1.75l) milk	3 oz (75 g) flour
1 large onion, peeled	12 oz (350 g) cheese, grated
4 bay leaves	salt and pepper
grated nutmeg	

Preheat oven: 400°F, 200°C; gas mark 6.

Cook and drain the pasta shells according to instructions on the packet. Lightly cook the broccoli until just tender, drain and roughly chop. In a saucepan bring the milk to the boil with the onion, bay leaves, grated nutmeg and peppercorns, then cover and leave to cool before straining.

Make a cheese sauce by melting the butter, stir in the flour and cook for 2–3 minutes. Gradually pour in the strained milk and bring to the boil, stirring constantly until the sauce thickens. Take off the heat and add 10 oz (300 g) grated cheese and season with salt and pepper.

Combine the pasta shells, broccoli and cheese sauce together and spoon into an ovenproof dish. Sprinkle on the balance of the cheese and bake in the oven for about 20 minutes or until golden and bubbling.

Serve with a tomato or green salad.

BREAD AND BUTTER PUDDING

8 slices of white bread, buttered	4 eggs
2 tablespoons (30 ml) demerara sugar	$1\frac{1}{4}$ pts (675 ml) milk
4 oz (125 g) sultanas	ground nutmeg

Preheat oven: 350°F, 180°C; gas mark 4.

Grease a 2–$2\frac{1}{2}$ pint (1.25–1.5 l) ovenproof dish. Cut the bread and butter slices in half and arrange, buttered side up, in layers in the ovenproof dish, sprinkling the layers with the sugar and sultanas. Finish with a layer of bread and sugar. Whisk the eggs lightly and add to the milk. Pour the whole lot over the bread, sprinkle some freshly grated nutmeg on top and bake in the oven for 30–40 minutes until set and lightly brown. Serve warm.

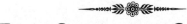

CRISPY CRUMBLE FRUIT PIE

8 oz (225 g) brown flour
8 oz (225 g) porridge oats
4 oz (125 g) butter
8 oz (225 g) light brown sugar

1 egg
little water
1½ lb (675 g) cooked fruits

Preheat oven: 350°F, 180°C; gas mark 4.

Suggested fruits are apple, blackberries, rhubarb, gooseberries, plums, etc., simmered with a scant amount of water and sugar to taste until barely tender. A little cinnamon would go particularly well with apples and plums as would ground ginger with rhubarb.

In a mixing bowl place the flour and porridge oats, then add the butter and rub in lightly using your finger tips. When it all looks crumbly and the fat evenly dispersed, add the sugar and combine well. Mix the egg with half of this mixture, together with a little water, to form a dough. Press into the base and sides of a 3 pint (1.75 l) pie dish. Fill with the cooked fruit of your choice and sprinkle on the balance of the crumble. Bake in the oven for 30–40 minutes until the topping is tinged with brown.

DATE, ORANGE AND CINNAMON FLAPJACK PUDDING

8 oz (225 g) dates, chopped
orange juice
pinch of cinnamon
6 oz (175 g) butter

2 tablespoons (30 ml) syrup
8 oz (225 g) porridge oats
4 oz (125 g) soft, light brown sugar
4 oz (125 g) plain wholemeal flour

Preheat oven: 375°F, 190°C; gas mark 5.

Grease a 7 × 7 in (18 × 18 cm) tin. In a saucepan cook the dates with enough orange juice to make a spreading consistency together with a pinch of cinnamon. Melt together the butter and syrup and combine together with all the dry ingredients. Press half this mixture into the greased tin, spread over the dates and cover with the remaining mixture. Bake in the oven for 20–25 minutes until just browning.

Serve cold in slices or warm as a pudding with some cream.

WARWICKSHIRE APPLE CAKE

1 lb (450 g) self-raising flour
½ teaspoon (2.5 ml) mixed spices
½ teaspoon (2.5 ml) nutmeg
pinch of salt
6 oz (175 g) sultanas
6 oz (175 g) Granny Smith apples,
    finely chopped

8 oz (225 g) soft margarine
8 oz (225 g) caster sugar
2 eggs
¼ pt (150 ml) milk
1 Granny Smith apple, sliced
1 tablespoon (15 ml) demerara sugar

Preheat oven: 350°F, 180°C; gas mark 4.

Grease and line a 9 in (23 cm) cake tin. Sift together the flour, spices, nutmeg and salt and stir in the sultanas and chopped apples. In a large mixing bowl cream together the soft margarine and caster sugar until light and fluffy. Gradually beat in the eggs (don't worry if the mixture should curdle slightly). Gently stir in the flour, spices and fruit and pour in the milk to make a stiffish mixture. Spoon into the cake tin and smooth out the top. Brush the top with water and lay the apple slices in a circle. Brush once again with water and sprinkle on the demerara sugar. Bake in the oven for approximately 1¼ hours. Cool slightly before turning out on to a wire rack.

Scurvy

Scurvy has long been recognised as an affliction of the poor and sailors deprived of fresh food on long voyages (see p. 30). But now it has been argued by Susan Maclean Kybett, Fellow of the Royal Historical Society, that the highest and mightiest in the land were similarly afflicted. Henry VIII, his daughters Mary and Elizabeth, and his colossally wealthy prelate, Cardinal Wolsey, all manifested symptoms of scurvy. Meat formed the mainstay of a privileged diet, while fresh fruit and vegetables were regarded as more suitable for peasants. One prominent physician warned that fruit 'do ingender ylle humours and be ofteytimes the cause of putrified fevers'. If the King suffered from dietary malnutrition, then it is more than probable that most of his courtiers did too.

CHIRK CASTLE

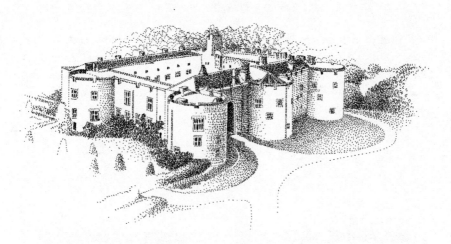

O N THE borders, 'the marches' between England and Wales, Edward
I organised a chain of castles to be built to consolidate his
conquests against the Welsh. Chirk Castle was begun in 1295 by
Roger Mortimer, on land confiscated from Llywelyn ap Gruffydd ap
Madog – 'the dragon of Chirk with the obstinate spear'. As visitors approach
through immense wrought-iron gates, up a long drive and then climb a
steep hill under the huge, stone-block walls and drum towers of the
forbidding entrance, it is not difficult to imagine the turbulent medieval
history of Chirk. Many of its owners were powerful political figures and
most of them met untimely ends.

Although life at Chirk is now more tranquil, on each side of the great
internal courtyard you can taste the lives of previous inhabitants of the
castle. Adam's Tower is medieval: below the guardroom is a damp, evoca-
tively nasty dungeon; above is a series of small rooms equipped with
accurately placed 'murder holes' in the floors. The Magistrates' Court is a
narrow chamber with a charming rough-cut frieze, the only plasterwork to
survive the Civil War. Chirk, then owned by Sir Thomas Myddelton, was
besieged and sacked during the war, but the family returned to restore the
castle, and their descendants live here still.

The castle proper is entered on the north side. The Cromwell Hall feels
seventeenth century but was in fact created by the Victorian architect A. W.
Pugin. A graceful staircase leads up to the eighteenth-century state rooms –
the State Dining Room, Saloon, Drawing Room and a 100-ft Long Gallery,
sumptuously furnished and hung with portraits by Kneller, Lely, Van Dyck
and others.

On the south side of the quadrangle is the Servants' Hall, dark but not depressing; servants ate here and a strict hierarchy determined who sat near the fire, who by the door and who was served first. On the walls are lively pictures of, amongst others, 'Welch Wilkes, Chirk Castle scullion' and a set of severe rules – 'No noise, no strife nor swear at all, But all be decent in the Hall.'

Good guidelines for today's visitors to observe in the tea-room in the delightful Old Kitchen opposite, where the tables in the area for booked parties are in circular turrets, with wonderful views. Here are interesting soups, good savoury tarts, a vegetable crumble that is a main-course variation on an old favourite.

Notes to servants that hang in the Servants' Hall at Chirk Castle:

SERVANTS' HALL
No noise, no strife nor swear at all
But all be decent in the Hall.

Rules to be Observed
That every servant must:
Take off his hat on entering here
Sit in proper place at table
Keep himself clean becoming his station
Shut the door after him
Drink in his turn

That no servant be:
Guilty of cursing or swearing
Telling tales
Speaking disrespectfully of anyone
Wasting meat or drink
Intermeddling with any other's business unless requested to assist

NB The person offending to be deprived his allowance of beer – for the first offence three days, second offence one whole month and more often his behaviour to be laid before Mr Myddelton.

CAULIFLOWER SOUP

2 oz (50 g) butter
1 large onion, chopped
2 lb (900 g) cauliflower, chopped
1 large potato, chopped

4 cups 1¾ pt (1 l) vegetable stock
salt and freshly ground black pepper
½ pt (250 ml) double cream
generous amount of parsley, chopped

In a large saucepan gently fry the chopped onion until transparent. Add the cauliflower, potato and vegetable stock, bring to the boil and simmer with a lid on for around 20 minutes or until the vegetables are tender. Take off the heat and cool slightly before blending in a food processor. Return to the pan and season with salt and pepper. Before serving pour in the double cream and garnish with chopped fresh parsley.

This recipe can be used to make celery or leek soup, substituting the cauliflower.

LEEK PIE

Pastry

4 oz (125 g) wholemeal flour
2 oz (50 g) plain flour
3 oz (75 g) Cheddar cheese, grated

3 oz (75 g) butter or margarine, chilled
1 egg yolk
cold water to mix

Filling

4 oz (125 g) butter or margarine
2 lb (900 g) leeks (sliced ½ in [1.25 cm] rounds)
4 oz (125 g) flour
¾ pt (400 ml) milk

rind and juice ½ lemon
pinch of ground nutmeg
2 oz (50 g) chopped hazelnuts
2 oz (50 g) raisins
salt and pepper

Preheat oven: 400°F, 200°C; gas mark 6.

Place the flours and grated cheese in a food processor together with the chilled butter and process for a few seconds until the mixture resembles coarse bread-crumbs. Take off the lid and add the egg yolk together with 1 tablespoon (15 ml) of cold water. Process until the mixture forms a ball around the central column. If this does not happen after a few seconds, take off the lid and add a little more water. Place in a plastic bag and leave to rest in the fridge while you make the filling.

Melt the butter in a large saucepan and sauté the chopped leeks gently until tender. Stir in the flour and cook over a gentle heat for 2 or 3 minutes.

59

Pour in the milk and bring to the boil, stirring all the time with a wooden spoon, until the sauce has thickened. Add all the remaining ingredients and season to taste. Place in an ovenproof pie dish. Roll out the pastry, cover the pie and brush with milk or beaten egg. Place in the oven and bake for 30 minutes.

This pie has a particularly tasty filling.

VEGETABLE CRUMBLE

Crumble Topping
4 oz (125 g) butter _hard_ _marge_

6 oz (175 g) wholemeal flour

3 oz _whole wheat_
3 oz _"   " w/ bran_

6 oz (175 g) mature Cheddar cheese, grated

2 oz (50 g) chopped walnuts

Vegetable Base
1 lb 12 oz (800 g) mixed vegetables —
   such as potatoes, carrots, parsnips,
   leeks and mushrooms

1 large onion, chopped

2 oz (50 g) butter

1 oz (25 g) wholemeal flour

small tin chopped tomatoes

$\frac{1}{4}$ pt (150 ml) vegetable stock

$\frac{1}{2}$ pt (250 ml) milk

a good handful of chopped parsley

salt and freshly ground black pepper

Preheat oven: 375°F, 190°C; gas mark 5.

Rub the butter into the flour until the mixture resembles fine crumbs. Add the cheese, nuts and some black pepper to taste and combine well.

Chop all the vegetables and in a large saucepan melt the butter and sauté the onion until transparent. Add the prepared vegetables and cook over a gentle heat, stirring occasionally, for 10–15 minutes. Take off the heat, stir in the flour and the remaining ingredients. Bring to the boil and simmer for 15–20 minutes until the vegetables are just tender. Transfer to a large ovenproof dish and press the crumble topping over the vegetables. Bake in the oven for 30–40 minutes. Garnish with a little parsley.

COUNTRY CHEESE TART
WITH GARLIC AND FRESH HERBS

Pastry

4 oz (125 g) plain wholewheat flour
2 oz (50 g) self-raising flour
pinch of salt

2 oz (50 g) margarine
2 oz (50 g) vegetarian lard
cold water

Filling

1 oz (25 g) butter
2 oz (50 g) onion, finely chopped
2 cloves garlic, chopped
3 eggs, lightly beaten
¼ pt (150 ml) milk
¼ pt (150 ml) double cream

freshly chopped herbs of your choice
3 oz (75 g) mature Welsh Cheddar
  cheese
salt and pepper
2 tomatoes, chopped
parsley, chopped

Preheat oven: 400°F, 200°C; gas mark 6.

Place the flours and salt in a mixing bowl, then cut the fats into small cubes and add to the bowl. Using your fingertips, gently rub the fat into the flour. When the mixture looks crumbly start to sprinkle in around 2 tablespoons (30 ml) of water. Gradually work this in with a knife, then draw together to form a ball with your hands. Place the pastry in a polythene bag and refrigerate for 20 minutes.

Roll out the pastry and line an 8 in (20 cm) flan tin. Melt the butter in a saucepan and gently sauté the chopped onion and garlic until lightly brown. Cool for a few minutes before spreading over the pastry case. Place the eggs, milk, cream, herbs and cheddar cheese in a bowl, beat until well mixed and season with salt and pepper. Pour the mixture over the onions and sprinkle with chopped tomatoes and fresh parsley. Place the flan on a baking sheet in the oven and bake for 30–40 minutes until golden brown (reduce heat and cook for a further 5–10 minutes if the egg mixture is not quite set).

Stilton and Celery Tart
(an alternative filling)

As for Country Cheese Tart but substitute 3 oz (75 g) of blue Stilton cheese for the 3 oz (75 g) mature Welsh Cheddar and add 8 oz (225 g) very thinly sliced celery, simmered in a little butter until tender and then drained (omit the herbs, garlic and tomatoes).

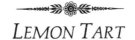

LEMON TART

Pastry (pâté sucre)

4 oz (125 g) plain flour

pinch of salt

3 oz (75 g) butter (straight from the
    fridge)

1 oz (25 g) caster sugar

1 egg yolk

1 tablespoon (15 ml) cold water

Filling

8 oz (225 g) caster sugar

8 oz (225 g) butter

4 eggs, lightly beaten

2 lemons – juice and grated rind

Preheat oven: 350°F, 180°C; gas mark 4

Combine the flour, salt, butter and sugar in a food processor and process until the mixture resembles coarse bread-crumbs. Add the egg yolk and 1 tablespoon (15 ml) cold water and continue to process until the mixture forms a ball around the central column. Do not overprocess – stop the machine as soon as the ball has formed. Place the pastry into a plastic bag and leave to rest in the fridge (around 20 minutes) while you make the filling.

Roll out the pastry and line an 8 in (20 cm) flan tin. In a saucepan melt together the caster sugar and butter. Take off the heat and stir in the lightly beaten eggs, then the juice and rind of the lemons. Pour this mixture into the pastry case and place the flan tin in the oven on a baking sheet (this will ensure that the pastry base is firm and that the flan filling sets well). Bake for 30 minutes when the top should be a light golden brown.

This is without question, the best Lemon Tart I have ever tasted, hot or cold.

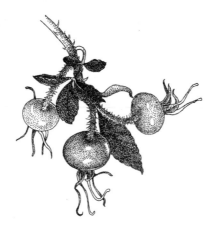

CLAREMONT
LANDSCAPE GARDEN

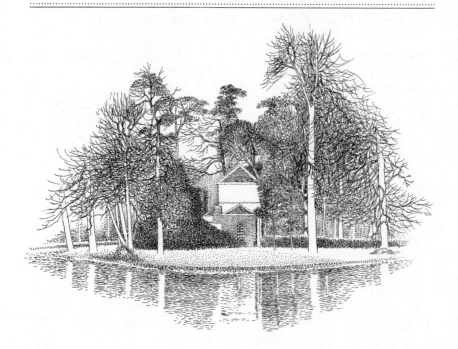

S PACE today is a luxury to be cherished, particularly in the built-up south-east of England. Claremont – 50 acres of spacious eighteenth-century landscape garden – is bounded on one side by the busy A307, the old trunk road from London to Portsmouth, and on all the other sides by the houses and gardens of prosperous suburbia.

The landscape garden is a distinctly English contribution to the history of gardening – a reaction to the earlier, formal planning and planting. In landscape gardens, park and garden merge imperceptibly into a harmonious whole, nature is respected and enhanced rather than rigidly moulded to a pattern. Flowers play a minor role; water, trees, and antique buildings are more important.

At Claremont, all these pleasures can be experienced; the reflection of trees on water, the impressive amphitheatre, a ruined grotto for melancholy thoughts, an elegant island pavilion. Black swans and myriad duck float on the lake which also contains huge slow-moving carp.

This garden, so peaceful now, has had a chequered history. Many owners and gardeners have altered and influenced Claremont, amongst them Sir John Vanbrugh, Charles Bridgeman, William Kent, Lancelot 'Capability'

Brown, Lord Clive of India and Prince Leopold of Saxe-Coburg, Queen Victoria's uncle. By 1976 the garden was a 'lake within a wood', the grotto decayed, the amphitheatre invisible and the original planting obscured beneath self-sown birch and scrub. Restoration meant stripping back layers of undergrowth to reveal the lovely garden we enjoy today, not one man's creation but the essence of the English Landscape Garden, art and nature combined to form a succession of contrasts for the onlooker's pleasure.

A right turn at the entrance to the garden takes one to the tea-room, newly built in a rustic style of which William Kent would have approved. Peacocks scratch outside, inside you will find imaginative, interesting food, far outside the usual scope of a tea-room. Salamongundy is eighteenth-century, a vegetarian version an imaginative twentieth-century idea. Indian pancakes and carrot pudding provide a delicate compliment to one of Claremont's famous owners, Clive of India.

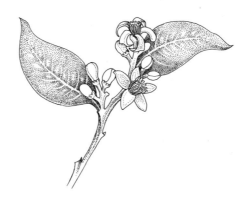

Shaw's Corner
George Bernard Shaw, whose house, Shaw's Corner at Ayot St Lawrence, is now owned by the National Trust, was a fervent vegetarian who lived to 94. He was vigorous in his vegetarian logic: 'The strongest animals such as the bull are vegetarian. Look at me, I have ten times as much health and energy as a meat eater.... My hearse will be followed not by mourning coaches but by herds of oxen, sheep, swine, flocks of poultry and a small travelling aquarium of live fish, all wearing white scarves in honour of the man who perished rather than eat his fellow creatures.'

SPRING SOUP

1 large onion	1 bunch of nettle tops
2 sticks of celery	1 bunch of watercress
2 carrots	1 bunch of dandelion leaves
2 tomatoes	1 lb (450 g) spinach or sorrel
1 bayleaf	salt and pepper
pinch of thyme	thick cream to serve
4 pt (2.50 l) water	

Sauté in a large pan with a little butter or oil the chopped onion, celery, carrots, tomatoes, bayleaf and thyme. When softened add 4 pints (2.50 l) of water, bring to the boil and simmer for half an hour. Strain the stock (or if you would like a more substantial soup, leave the stock ingredients) and add all the leaf mixtures. Reheat and as soon as they have turned dark green and wilted, liquidise in a blender or processor. Heat before serving and add some thick cream.

This must be made early in the year before young growth becomes tough and woody.

SALAMONGUNDY

More of a concept than a recipe – in 1747 Mrs Hannah Glasse wrote, 'you may always make Salamongundy of such things as you have, according to your fancy'.

Salamongundy is basically an English composite salad, similar to the Mediterranean Salade Niçoise. Originally it consisted of cold meats combined with lettuce, grapes and anchovies but there are many variations.

In this vegetarian version the base consists of a mixture of colourful and tasty leaves such as curly endive, cos, lollo rosso, oakleaf, young dandelion leaves, spinach – whatever is available. A layer is placed on a large flat dish, then other vegetables are layered or piled on top to make a colourful display. You can use: leeks and mushrooms cooked 'à la grecque' in a little vinegar and olive oil and cooled; tiny new potatoes cooked and dressed with walnut oil and mint; raw carrot with a poppy-seed dressing; blanched green beans, etc. Hard-boiled eggs can also be added and there should always be a fruit element such as chopped red apples or grapes.

Place the dish in the centre of the table and let your guests help themselves. Served with a good selection of bread and a bottle of Alsace Gewurztraminer, it makes a perfect summer lunch or supper.

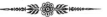

RICE AND CHICKPEA FLOUR PANCAKES WITH AN INDIAN SPICED STUFFING

Pancakes

2 oz (50 g) besan flour (Gram flour) –
  available from Indian foodstores or
  health food shops
2 oz (50 g) ground rice

approximately 8 fl oz (225 ml) milk
1 egg, lightly beaten
salt and pepper

Filling

1 large onion
2 tablespoons (30 ml) oil
1 teaspoon (5 ml) whole cumin
1 teaspoon (5 ml) kalonji (onion seeds
  or nigella)

2 teaspoons (10 ml) Madras curry
  paste
2 lb (900 g) waxy potatoes
14 oz (400 g) tin tomatoes
2 oz (50 g) frozen peas
salt and pepper

Sift the besan flour into a bowl. Add the ground rice and mix to a paste with a little of the milk. Mix in the beaten egg and the balance of the milk to make a pouring batter. Season and allow to rest for approximately 20 minutes.

Fry the pancakes in a non-stick frying pan or with the addition of a little oil and, as each one is done, stack on a plate and keep covered in a low oven.

To make the filling, fry the chopped onion in oil, add cumin and kalonji and continue to sauté for a few minutes. Mix in the curry paste and potatoes which have been peeled and cut into approximately 1 in (2.5 cm) cubes. Pour in the tin of tomatoes and add a little water, if necessary, to cover. Put on a lid and simmer until the potatoes are done (but still firm). Raise the heat and cook uncovered until the sauce is thick, stirring frequently. Add the frozen peas and salt and pepper to taste.

Place an equal amount of filling on each pancake and roll up. Serve with a coconut relish made by soaking desiccated coconut in milk for an hour, draining and then adding chopped cucumbers and fresh parsley or coriander or natural yoghurt with the addition of some freshly chopped mint.

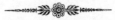

TOMATO AND BASIL TART
WITH OLIVE OIL PASTRY

Pastry

1 clove of garlic, crushed
5 tablespoons (75 ml) olive oil
1 tablespoon (15 ml) water

6 oz (175 g) plain flour
1 teaspoon (5 ml) salt

Filling

1 large onion
3 tablespoons (45 ml) olive oil
3 lb (1.4kg) tomatoes

1 bunch of fresh basil, chopped
1 teaspoon (5 ml) sugar
salt and pepper

Preheat oven: 400°F, 200°C; gas mark 6.

Fry the garlic in oil and allow to cool a little before adding the water (the oil will spit if too hot). Beat into the flour and salt and form the mixture into a ball. It is not possible to roll this pastry in the traditional way. However, it can either be rolled between two sheets of greaseproof paper or pressed into an 8 in (20 cm) loose-bottomed flan tin, using fingertips. Chill for approximately 20 minutes. Bake blind in the oven for 15–20 minutes.

Lower oven heat to: 350°F, 180°C; gas mark 4.

To make the filling, chop the onion finely and sauté in the oil for a minute or two. Skin and de-seed the tomatoes, place in the pan and cook until reduced to a thick pulp. Add half of the basil, sugar and salt and pepper to taste and spoon into the baked flan case. Bake in a low oven for about half an hour. Just before serving sprinkle with the remaining basil and serve with a green salad and crusty bread.

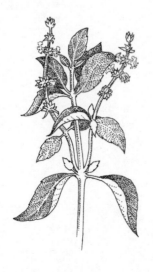

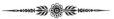

APPLE AND STILTON STRUDEL

1 large packet strudel pastry (filo
   pastry)
4 tablespoons (60 ml) vegetable oil
1 lb (450 g) Stilton cheese

5 Granny Smith apples
4 oz (125 g) fresh white bread-crumbs
2 tablespoons (30 ml) melted butter

Preheat oven: 400°F, 200°C; gas mark 6.

Defrost the packet of strudel pastry and lay out five rectangular sheets with the short edge nearest you. Brush each sheet with vegetable oil before laying on the next. Crumble the Stilton over the pastry, leaving a small gap at either end and at the sides. Peel and chop the apples and cut into chunks. Spread on top of the cheese and sprinkle over a good handful of fresh bread-crumbs. Starting at the edge nearest you, roll up the strudel as tightly as possible without breaking the pastry. Place on a greased baking sheet with the edges down. Brush with melted butter and sprinkle on the balance of the bread-crumbs. Bake in the oven for approximately 30 minutes.

    Cut into large slices and serve as a lunch or supper dish with a salad of your choice.

CARROT HALWA

$1\frac{1}{2}$ lb (675 g) carrots, peeled and finely
   grated
4 oz (125 g) unsalted butter
6 cardamon pods
2 oz (50 g) sultanas

6 oz (175 g) caster sugar
2 oz (50 g) ground almonds
2 tablespoons (30 ml) honey
14 oz (400 g) can condensed milk
a few drops of almond essence

Cover the grated carrots with water and cook gently until soft. Drain well and return the carrots to the saucepan, then add all the other ingredients and cook gently until the mixture is quite thick. Press the mixture into a baking tray so that it is about $1\frac{1}{2}$ in (3.75 cm) in depth. Cool and then refrigerate until required. Serve with single cream in small squares as a pudding.

    This pudding is extremely rich and has a subtle, delicate flavour.

CLIVEDEN

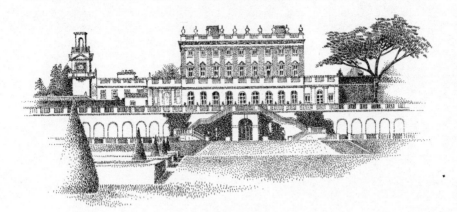

IGH up above the Thames in Buckinghamshire stands Cliveden, an Italianate villa built in the mid-nineteenth century. It is the third house to have been built on the site, the first two having been destroyed by fire. The present house was built in 1850–1 to the design of Sir Charles Barry for the 2nd Duke of Sutherland. It was during the early years of the nineteenth century, when the first house was a ruin, that the great statesman George Canning is thought to have spent hours beneath the oak tree that now bears his name. The view of the Thames from beneath its branches is one of the most famous on the river.

The house is now used as an hotel, but the visitor can stand on the immense south-facing terrace, look down over the Borghese balustrade and across the clipped conical yews and geometrically planted beds of the parterre to the river far below and the rolling hills beyond. The 1st Lord Astor, who bought the house in 1893, laid out the Long Garden and the delightful water garden with its irregular ponds full of carp, stepping stones and a pagoda. He also filled the grounds with statuary, including Roman marble sarcophagi, and built the huge Fountain of Love to the north of the house.

When his eldest son, Waldorf, married the Virginian beauty Nancy Langhorne in 1906, Lord Astor gave them the house. As Lady Astor, Nancy became the first female Member of Parliament to take her seat, and between the wars she made Cliveden a centre of political and literary society. A woman of strongly held views, she detested the consumption of alcohol and enjoyed several famous verbal duels with Sir Winston Churchill on the subject. She was also a firm Christian Scientist, and although she herself enjoyed good health, her opposition to orthodox medical treatment could bring problems to her friends and family.

After a walk in the grounds at Cliveden, visit the National Trust restaurant in the white-painted conservatory on the east side of the house. Cliveden is one of only two properties that I have included in both my collections of Trust recipes. I make no apologies; Maureen Smith is a superb vegetarian cook, and her recipes are imaginative and unusual. Here are three vegetable pâtés and five interesting hot dishes, including a spicy vegetables and rice, which Maureen invented to tempt jaded appetites during a heatwave.

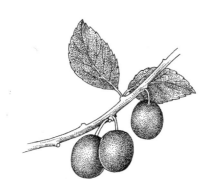

Lentil and Wine Pâté

12 oz (350 g) red lentils
1½ pt (750 ml) red wine
2 oz (50 g) butter
2 large onions, chopped
4 oz (125 g) carrots, finely chopped
2 sticks celery, finely chopped

2 cloves of garlic, crushed
2 teaspoons (10 ml) dried herbs
4 oz (125 g) ground mixed nuts
4 oz (125 g) cheese, grated
2 eggs, lightly beaten
salt and pepper

Preheat oven: 350°F, 180°C; gas mark 4.

Prepare a 2 lb (900 g) loaf tin by lining the base and sides with silicon paper. Place the lentils and red wine in a saucepan, bring to the boil and simmer for 20 minutes until the lentils are tender and the liquid absorbed. In a large saucepan melt the butter and fry the onions, carrot, celery and garlic for approximately 10 minutes when they should be softened and light brown. Take off the heat and add the cooked lentils, herbs, nuts, cheese and eggs. Mix everything together and season with salt and pepper. Spoon the mixture into the prepared tin and cover with a piece of foil. Bake in the oven for around 1¼ hours, removing the foil for the last 15 minutes. Allow to rest for a while to firm up the pâté before very carefully turning out and removing the lining paper.

This pâté can be served either hot or cold, decorated with fresh herbs.

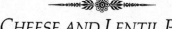

CHEESE AND LENTIL PÂTÉ

1 lb (450 g) red lentils
1 oz (25 g) butter
2 large onions, finely chopped
1 clove of garlic, crushed

8 oz (225 g) cheese, grated
handful chopped fresh parsley
4 eggs, lightly beaten
salt and pepper

Preheat oven: 350°F, 180°C; gas mark 4.

Prepare a 2 lb (900 g) loaf tin by lining the base and sides with silicon paper. In a large saucepan place the lentils with just enough water to cover. Bring to the boil and simmer until the lentils are cooked and have absorbed all the water. This will take around 20 minutes. While they are cooking melt the butter in a small frying pan and gently sauté the finely chopped onions and crushed garlic until transparent. Add to the cooked lentils together with the grated cheese, parsley and eggs. Season well with salt and pepper and spoon into the loaf tin. Bake in the oven for $1\frac{1}{4}$ hours. Leave to cool before turning out and removing the lining paper.

Serve this pâté cold with a salad.

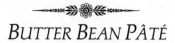

BUTTER BEAN PÂTÉ

8 oz (225 g) dried butter beans
2 cloves of garlic, crushed
juice $\frac{1}{2}$ lemon
$\frac{1}{4}$ pt (150 ml) double cream

salt and freshly ground black pepper
freshly chopped parsley
1 tablespoon (15 ml) spring onions,
   finely chopped

Soak the beans overnight, drain and cook in fresh water until they are very tender. Drain and allow to cool. Place the beans in a food processor together with the garlic, lemon juice and double cream and process until the mixture is almost smooth (if you wish you can also have a more coarse texture). Season with salt and pepper and stir in the parsley and chopped spring onions. Pack into individual ramekins and chill until required (it will keep well in a fridge).

Serve with crispy bread. Makes an excellent starter or serve with salads as a light main course.

LEEK AND MUSHROOM CROUSTADE

Base

3 oz (75 g) fresh bread-crumbs

4 oz (125 g) mixed chopped nuts

1 teaspoon (5 ml) dried mixed herbs (or fresh if you have them)

2 oz (50 g) butter

salt and pepper

Topping

2 oz (50 g) butter

1 large onion, chopped

1 tablespoon (15 ml) flour

$\frac{1}{2}$–$\frac{3}{4}$ pt (250–400 ml) milk

6 oz (175 g) cheese, grated

12 oz (350 g) leeks, cooked and sliced

8 oz (225 g) mushrooms, slightly cooked

salt and pepper

Preheat oven: 350°F, 180°C; gas mark 4.

Mix together all the ingredients for the base, season well with salt and pepper and press into the base of an 8 in (20 cm) loose-bottomed flan tin. Bake in the oven for 15 minutes until golden brown and crisp.

Melt the butter in a saucepan and fry the onion until transparent. Stir in the flour and cook for a minute or two before pouring in the milk. Stirring all the time, bring to the boil, then add 4 oz of the grated cheese, cooked leeks and mushrooms. Season with salt and pepper and spoon on top of the croustade. Sprinkle on the balance of the cheese and return the croustade to the oven and bake for around 20 minutes. Leave to cool slightly to give the mixture time to set before taking out of the tin.

Tastes good both lukewarm and cold!

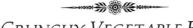

CRUNCHY VEGETABLE BAKE

1 large onion

1 green pepper

1 red pepper

8 oz (225 g) mushrooms

3–4 sticks of celery

2 tablespoons (30 ml) oil

6 oz (175 g) fresh brown bread-crumbs

4 oz (125 g) cheese, grated

herbs of your choice (optional)

1 large egg, lightly beaten

salt and freshly ground pepper

Topping

2 oz (50 g) bread-crumbs

2 oz (50 g) cheese, grated

salt and pepper

Preheat oven: 350°F, 180°C; gas mark 4.

If this dish is to be served hot it is important to chop all the vegetables very finely so that the loaf will hold its shape when turned out. This is not so essential when serving it cold.

Prepare a large loaf tin by lining the base and sides with silicon paper. Wash and chop all the vegetables and fry in oil in a large saucepan, stirring and tossing frequently until just tender. Take off the heat and cool a little before adding the bread-crumbs, grated cheese and lightly beaten egg. Season well with salt and freshly ground black pepper. Spoon the mixture into the loaf tin and make the topping.

Mix the two ingredients of the topping together and season with salt and pepper. Gently press on top of the vegetable mixture and bake in the oven for 40–50 minutes until the topping is crisp and lightly browned.

If serving hot, turn out very carefully on to a plate and peel off the lining. Place a serving dish gently on top of the loaf and turn over so that the topping is now, where it should be, on the top.

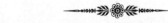

BUTTER BEAN AND LEEK BAKE

6 oz (175 g) dried butter beans	2 large onions, chopped
½ pt (250 ml) milk	2 cloves of garlic, crushed
3 leeks, sliced and cooked	1 oz (25 g) flour
2 oz (50 g) butter	freshly chopped parsley

Topping
Use the topping for Crunchy Vegetable
   Bake, p.72.

Preheat oven: 375°F, 190°C; gas mark 5.

Soak and cook the butter beans in water until soft. Drain and reserve their liquid. Make their liquid up to ¾ pt (400 ml) with the milk. Cook the leeks in a little boiling water until tender and drain well. Melt the butter in a saucepan and gently sauté the onion and garlic until transparent. Stir in the flour and cook for a further minute or two before adding the milk mixture. Bring to the boil, stirring all the time, until the sauce thickens. Combine with the cooked leeks and plenty of chopped fresh parsley, and season with salt and pepper. Divide into 4 in (10 cm) ramekins, lightly press on the topping and bake in the oven for 20 minutes until the top is crisp and golden.

In the summer these individual ramekins can be served with a side salad or in the winter with a jacket potato.

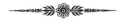

SPICED VEGETABLES AND RICE

1 lb (450 g) brown rice, cooked in
    vegetable stock
2 onions, finely chopped
2 teaspoons (10 ml) turmeric
2 cloves of garlic, crushed
2 oz (50 g) butter
1 large green pepper, chopped
6 oz (175 g) carrots, finely diced

4 oz (125 g) halved button mushrooms
pinch each of cinnamon, ginger and
    Chinese 5 spice
2 oz (50 g) split toasted almonds
1 oz (25 g) sesame seeds, toasted
2 oz (50 g) sultanas
salt and pepper
plenty of chopped parsley

In a large saucepan, fry the finely chopped onion, turmeric and garlic in the butter. Add the pepper, carrots, mushrooms and spices and continue to cook over a low heat until the vegetables are just tender. Stir frequently with a wooden spoon. Cool the mixture before adding the almonds, sesame seeds and sultanas and season with salt and pepper. Very carefully fold this mixture into the cooked rice together with the chopped parsley, then turn out on to a large serving dish. It can be served either hot or cold.

Maureen Smith invented this recipe during a heatwave; it is light but spicy to tickle jaded palates.

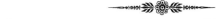

MUSHROOM AND BROAD BEAN GOUGÈRE

Choux pastry

4 oz (125 g) butter
10 fl oz (300 ml) water
5 oz (150 g) plain flour

4 eggs, lightly beaten
5 oz (150 g) cheese, grated
salt and pepper

Filling

3 oz (75 g) butter
2 oz (50 g) plain flour
$\frac{3}{4}$ pt (400 ml) milk
8 oz (225 g) fresh or frozen broad beans,
    cooked

8 oz (225 g) sliced mushrooms tossed in
    butter
salt and pepper

Preheat oven: 425°F, 220°C; gas mark 7.

Place the butter and water in a saucepan and heat gently until the butter has melted, then bring to the boil. Remove from the heat and add the flour all at once, beating well with a wooden spoon. Return the pan to a low heat and continue beating for around a minute until you have a smooth ball of paste that leaves the sides of the saucepan clean. Beat in the eggs a little at a time until you have a smooth glossy paste. Add 4 oz (125 g) grated cheese and season with salt and pepper.

Spoon dessertspoonfuls of the mixture around the edge of a large shallow ovenproof dish, sprinkle on the remainder of the cheese and bake for about 40 minutes, until the gougère is puffed up and golden brown.

For the filling make a parsley sauce: melt the butter in a saucepan, stir in the flour and cook for a minute or two before pouring in the milk. Stirring all the time, bring to the boil, then add a generous amount of parsley. Fold in the cooked vegetables and spoon into the centre of the gougère when you remove it from the oven (if there is any over serve it separately) and serve straight away.

Belton's Exercise Chair

In the Library at Belton is an exercise chair made for Lord Tyrconnel in 1754. Although spritely in his youth, by this time the Viscount was sixty-four and beyond active equestrianism. With its bellows-type action, the chair gave him some small reminder of his riding days.

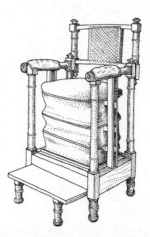

ERDDIG

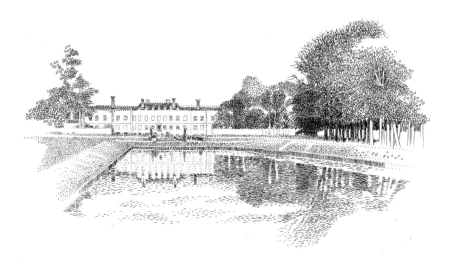

A PIOUS, temperate, sensible country gentleman' – Simon Yorke I died in 1767 but his epitaph perfectly describes the Simons and Philips (eldest Yorke sons were invariably christened with one of these names), squires of Erddig for the next two centuries. They were also antiquarians, conservationists and the best of employers, leaving a unique record in writing, pictures and photographs of their servants and their way of life.

At Erddig, visitors enter the house, appropriately, by the back door after an extensive and fascinating tour of the buildings necessary to the running of a large estate. Some are still in use; the joiners' shop and the smithy hum with activity. The Yorkes did not believe in obsolescence: in the stables and wagon shed are aged bicycles, a 1907 Rover, 1920s Austins and nineteenth-century estate carts that were still in use in 1930. Beyond the stables is the female servants' preserve, comprising bakehouse, wet laundry, dry laundry (still fitted with huge racks and mangles) and, finally, the hub of this busy world, the New (in 1774) Kitchen. The kitchen is a wonderful room painted a peculiar shade of blue against flies, the great windows overlooking the garden, reflecting the Yorkes' unusual concern for the well-being of their staff. This interest in the staff continues in the basement passage, which is lined with nineteenth-century photographs, each with an appropriate verse penned by Philip II. Past the housekeeper's room, the agent's office and the still-room lies the servants' hall, again lined with portraits, this time eighteenth- and early nineteenth-century paintings with verses by Simon II. The carpenter, woodman, housemaid, and even a negro coach-boy are celebrated here. On either side of the range are hatchments recording long-serving butlers.

And so at last, the green baize door is reached and above stairs.

Erddig is not a grand house, but the Yorkes loved it and filled it with treasures. Perhaps the grandest room is Thomas Hopper's Dining Room, lined with portraits of all the owners of Erddig since 1716 — except one. Here, and in the Saloon, Library, Entrance Hall and Drawing Room can be found fine furniture and china. Simon II, the missing owner, hangs in the delicate Chinese Room. Upstairs, the survival of the State Bed, despite a perilous eighteenth-century journey and neglect and rainwater in this century, is one of the wonders of Erddig. Now happily restored, its embroidery hangings glitter in a room lined with exquisite Chinese wall-paper. Upstairs, too, are little servants' rooms under the eaves of the house, a nursery full of toys, and a dark gallery adorned with eighteenth-century mother-of-pearl models created by Elizabeth Ratcliffe, an artistic lady's maid to Mrs Yorke.

Stroll in the formal garden, then climb the stairs to the restaurant in the old hay barn, often passing the delicious smell of freshly baked bread. Many interesting old recipes exist in the Erddig archives: the carrot soup now served at Erddig is a tasty adaptation, and others are reproduced here with more manageable quantities and instructions.

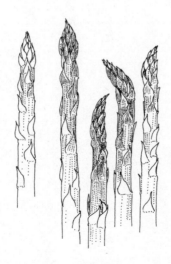

ASPARAGUS SOUP

1 bundle fresh asparagus (about 1 lb
[450 g])
4 oz (125 g) butter
1 small onion
$\frac{3}{4}$ pt (400 ml) vegetable stock

2 oz (50 g) flour
$\frac{3}{4}$ pt (400 ml) extra strong vegetable
stock (double strength)
salt and freshly ground black pepper
$\frac{1}{2}$ pt (250 ml) double cream

Remove the asparagus tips and reserve for garnishing. Cut off the tough ends, scrape the stems clean and cut these into 1 in (2.5 cm) pieces. Melt the butter, add the asparagus pieces and chopped onion and cook until barely tender, stirring regularly. Add the ordinary vegetable stock and simmer until the stalks are cooked and soft. Stir in the flour, add the double stock and continue stirring until the soup comes to the boil. Pour into a food processor and blend until smooth.

Steam or simmer very gently in water the asparagus tips until cooked but still crunchy.

Return the soup to the saucepan and just before serving reheat. Pour into individual bowls, swirl in some double cream to give a marble effect and scatter the asparagus tips on top.

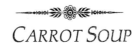

CARROT SOUP

1 lb (450 g) carrots
1 large onion
2 oz (50 g) butter
$2\frac{1}{2}$ pints (1.5 l) vegetable stock

$\frac{1}{2}$ teaspoon (2.5 ml) crushed coriander
2 tablespoons (30 ml) ground rice
juice of two oranges
salt and pepper

Slice the carrots and onions thinly and sweat with the butter in a large saucepan with the lid on until soft. Pour in the stock and crushed coriander, bring to the boil and simmer for 15 minutes. Add the ground rice and orange juice and continue to simmer for a further half an hour. Liquidise in a blender or food processor, return to the pan and season to taste.

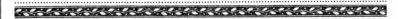

Broccoli Open Pie

SERVES EIGHT—TEN

10 oz (300 g) wholewheat pastry (use
  the pastry recipe from Chirk,
  Country Cheese Tart, p. 61)
6 oz (175 g) cheese, grated

2 lb (900 g) broccoli florets, blanched
  and drained
10 eggs
¾ pint (400 ml) double cream

Preheat oven: 425°F, 220°C; gas mark 7.

Line an 8 × 12 in (20 × 30.5 cm) ovenproof flan dish with the rolled out pastry. Cover the base with half the grated cheese. Evenly place the broccoli florets on top. Whisk the eggs until lightly beaten, add the double cream and continue to whisk until it is incorporated. Pour over the broccoli and sprinkle on the rest of the grated cheese. Bake in a hot oven for 45 minutes.

This is more than a light snack; it makes a substantial supper dish served with a salad or as part of a buffet. Chopped spinach could be used as an alternative to the broccoli.

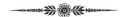

OLD ENGLISH BAKED RICE PUDDING

4 oz (125 g) pudding rice
rind of 1 lemon
1 pint (500 ml) milk
2 oz (50 g) caster sugar
4 eggs

2 oz (50 g) unsalted butter
2 oz (50 g) raisins
2 oz (50 g) sultanas
1 oz (25 g) chopped peel or glacé cherries
grated nutmeg

Preheat oven: 300°F, 150°C; gas mark 2.

In a large pan, bring plenty of water to the boil. Wash the rice, put this into the water and boil for 17 minutes exactly. Rinse the rice in a sieve under running cold water.

In a double boiler, infuse the lemon rind with the milk and sugar. Beat the eggs in a separate basin. Whisk in the hot milk and return the mixture to the pan, stirring all the time until the sauce coats the back of a spoon.

Take the pan off the heat (off the water, that is), add the butter, fruits and cold rice. Butter an ovenproof dish and pour the mixture into this. Stand the dish in a second dish or meat tin containing hot water. Grate a little nutmeg over the top and bake for half an hour or until the pudding is set.

If you wish, this can be served with pouring cream.

This old-fashioned recipe was recommended by the late Michael Smith.

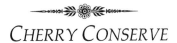

CHERRY CONSERVE

2 lb (900 g) dark red cherries
juice and rind of 2 lemons
1¾ lb (800 g) sugar with pectin

2–3 tablespoons (30–45 ml) cherry
brandy or kirsch

Stone the cherries and place them with the rind and lemon juice in a large, heavy-based saucepan. Simmer very gently for about 15 minutes or until really soft, stirring from time to time to prevent them from sticking. Add the sugar and stir over a low heat until dissolved. Increase the heat and boil rapidly until setting point is reached (approximately another 5 minutes). Stir in the alcohol of your choice, then ladle into the prepared jars and cover when cold with waxed discs and cellophane secured with rubber bands. Makes 3–4 lb (1.4–1.8 kg).

This makes a delicious, slightly runny conserve.

To Make a Rice Pudding

Take half a pound of rice and steep it in new milk a whole night, and in the morning drain the milk away, then take a quart of the sweetest cream and put the rice into it and boil it a little. Then sit it to cool an hour or two and put in the yolks of half a dozen eggs, a little clove and mace, currants and sugar, mix them well together, put in great store of suet, boil them and serve them after a day old.

c. 1685

To Preserve Cherries

Take of the best and fairest cherries. Take some two pound and with a pair of shears clip off their stalks by the middle then wash them clean and beware you bruise them not, then take of fine barbery sugar and set it over the fire with a quart of water. Let it seethe till it be something thick then put in your cherries and stir them together with a silver spoon and so let them boil always stirring and skimming them. To know when they be enough you must take up some of the syrup with one cherry and let it cool and if it is enough it will scarce run out. When they are cold put them up.

c. 1685

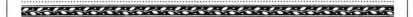

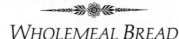

WHOLEMEAL BREAD

½ pint (250 ml) tepid water
1 teaspoon (5 ml) sugar
2 teaspoons (10 ml) dried yeast (½ oz
[12 g] fresh yeast)

1 lb (450 g) 100% wholemeal flour or
12 oz (350 g) wholewheat flour and
4 oz (100 g) strong plain white flour
1½ teaspoons (7.5 ml) salt
½ oz (12 g) vegetarian lard

Preheat oven: 400°F, 200°C; gas mark 6.

If using the dried yeast, place half the tepid water in a measuring jug and dissolve the sugar. Sprinkle the yeast over the top and leave in a warm place for 5–10 minutes until frothy (fresh yeast can be mixed in the water and used straightaway). Put the flour and salt into a mixing bowl and rub in the fat. Add the frothed-up yeast and the balance of the water and mix with a wooden spoon to give a fairly soft dough (add more water if necessary). Turn out on to a clean work surface and knead for 10 minutes until the dough is smooth and supple. Place in a well-greased 1 lb (450 g) loaf tin, pushing the dough well down into the corners and sides of the tin to encourage it to form a dome-shaped loaf. Put the tin in a warm place covered with a damp tea towel or placed in a lightly greased polythene bag, tied loosely, and leave to rise for 30–40 minutes or until the loaf has doubled in size and within $\frac{1}{4}$ in (6 mm) of the top of the bread tin.

If you wish, the surface of the loaf can be sprinkled with poppy seeds, sesame seeds, rolled oats or crack wheat. Brush the dough lightly with water or beaten egg to make the seeds stick.

Bake in the oven for about 40 minutes. Turn out the bread and, if cooked, the loaf will sound hollow when tapped underneath. Leave to cool on a wire tray.

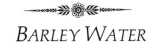

BARLEY WATER

2 oz (50 g) pearl barley
2 pints (1150 ml) water

2 lemons
sugar to taste

Wash the barley and put it to boil with the water and the thinly peeled rinds of the lemons. Boil very gently for 2 hours, then strain. Add sugar to taste, stir to dissolve it and leave to cool. Just before serving, add the juice from the 2 lemons.

Barley water was thought to be medicinal but there is no proof of this. However, as the old recipe suggests, it is a pleasantly cooling drink.

A Dainty Cooling Drink for a Hot Fever

Take French barley one ounce, boil it first in a quart of fair water a good while, then shift it and boil it in another quart of water a good while. Shift it again and boil it in a bottle of fair spring water to a quart, then take two ounces of sweet almonds, lay them to soak all night then stamp and strain them in the last barley water. Put to it 4 spoonsful of damask rose water, the juice of one lemon and with sugar sweeten it to your taste. Drink of this often when you are dry or hot.

c. 1685

KEDLESTON HALL

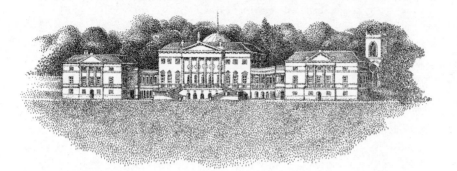

KEDLESTON HALL is one of the grandest houses in England. It was planned, built and furnished in the 1760s, the magnificent result of a collaboration between two young men, Nathaniel Curzon, 1st Lord Scarsdale and the Scottish architect Robert Adam. Tracing the plans of these two men takes one's breath away with the effrontery of the idea and scale of the task they took on, but probably older and more cautious men would not have achieved the splendid marriage between great house and great landscape that distinguishes Kedleston.

First, the old village was swept away and the highway moved. The canals and ponds were re-dug as lakes and cascades, the old formal gardens landscaped into the park. Visitors approach from the north up a long drive; as you cross the two lakes over an elegant three-arched bridge, the north front of the house appears before you, described as 'the grandest Palladian façade in Britain with few rivals anywhere in the world'. A dramatic portico dominates the central block, with great wings to left and right. It is an awe-inspiring sight. From the day he built the house, Lord Scarsdale opened the main rooms at Kedleston for visitors to admire. Today, visitors see the identical rooms, furnished and decorated to Adam's original designs. The Marble Hall and Saloon are the great receiving rooms, flanked on the one side by the arts – Music Room, Drawing Room and Library – and on the other by hospitality, the Dining Room and the principal apartment for important guests. The decoration is elaborate but not heavy in the pastel colours originally specified; Scarsdale's collection of pictures hang in the same spaces they were allotted in the original arrangement. Adam's furnishings can still arouse awe and admiration with his almost sensual use of gilt and rich silks. Huge pier glasses increase the architectural vistas.

Golden plumes crown the mirrors, while the state bed is a riot of palm trees and fronds. Most wonderful of all are the huge, blue, drawing-room sofas made for Adam by the cabinetmaker John Linnell, and supported by voluptuous tritons and sea-nymphs. Here, too, is evidence of young Adam's confidence, coupled with his Scot's concern for extravagance: the gold decorations on the skirting and dado stop behind the sofas and the walls are not painted behind the pictures. It would be no surprise to Adam to find everything in its place two centuries later.

Curzons have lived at Kedleston since the twelfth century and their portraits line the walls of the Family Corridor, together with pedigrees proudly showing their descent from Norman times. More Curzons can be seen in the answering Kitchen Corridor. Descending the Grand Staircase leads to an oriental museum housing the collection built up by Lord Curzon while Viceroy of India from 1899 to 1905.

Through the shop and along the Trophy Corridor lies the Great Kitchen, '48 feet by 24 feet and very lofty' noted Sir Christopher Sykes in 1794. Here, below a gallery supported on fine Doric columns, lunches and teas – speciality local Derby scones – are served on the original four huge scrubbed kitchen tables. Robert Adam would have approved of the motto 'Waste not, Want not' – over the giant range and spit. Cheese and onion bread, baked on the premises, is an unusual and interesting accompaniment to soup on a cold day, and salads on a warm one.

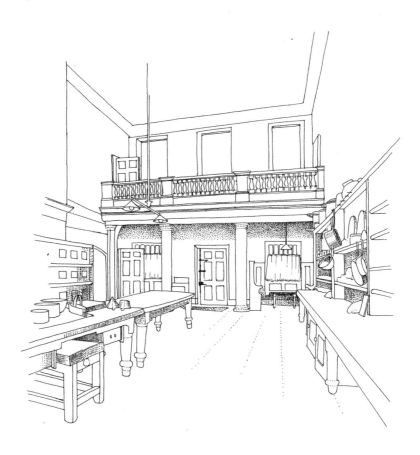

In the park at Kedleston, Robert Adam designed for Nathaniel Curzon two bath-houses. The first stands on the north shore of the middle lake. It was intended as a miniature spa, to be used by the public who came to Kedleston both to take the waters and to view the house. So many came that Adam designed an inn on the new turnpike road outside the park for their accommodation.

The second bath lies within the exquisite Fishing Room that Adam built in 1770 on the upper lake – a superb site for an invigorating dip.

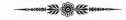

COUNTRY VEGETABLE SOUP

1 oz (25 g) butter	*1 lb (450 g) potatoes*
2 red peppers, chopped	*milk (optional)*
4 oz (125 g) peas (frozen)	*salt and pepper*
4 oz (125 g) carrots, sliced	*freshly chopped parsley*
4 oz (125 g) swede, chopped	*a few spring onion tops, chopped*
4 oz (125 g) sweetcorn	

The weights for vegetables are just a guide line – you need to end up with $1\frac{1}{2}$ lb (700 g) vegetables (excluding potatoes).

In a saucepan melt the butter and sweat all the vegetables, except the potatoes, until cooked. Peel the potatoes and barely cover them with water and boil until soft. Drain, reserving the cooking liquid, and mash until creamy. Return to the saucepan with the cooking liquid and vegetables and stir together. Thin if necessary with milk. Season with salt and pepper, reheat and serve piping hot, sprinkled with parsley and a few chopped onion tops.

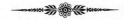

MUSHROOMS AND RED WINE SAUCE

2 oz (50 g) butter	$\frac{1}{4}$ *pint (150 ml) extra rich vegetable*
1 lb (450 g) button mushrooms – halves	*stock*
or quarters according to size	*scant $\frac{1}{4}$ pt (150 ml) red wine*
3 tomatoes	*salt and freshly ground black pepper*

Melt the butter in a saucepan and cook the mushrooms for a minute or two, stirring frequently. Skin, de-seed and chop the tomatoes and add to the mushrooms with the balance of the ingredients. Simmer together for around 5 minutes, then take out approximately half the sauce and blend it in a food processor. Return the sauce to the pan and simmer with the mushroom mixture for another 10 minutes. Makes about $\frac{1}{2}$ pint (250 ml).

This is a rich sauce, perfect to accompany the Lentil and Wine Pâté from Cliveden, p. 70 or the Minty Nut Loaf from Castle Drogo, p. 46.

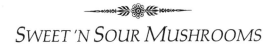

SWEET 'N SOUR MUSHROOMS

TO FILL FOUR RAMEKINS

12 oz (350 g) button mushrooms
1 oz (25 g) butter
1 dessertspoon (10 ml) creamed
  horseradish

1 teaspoon (5 ml) redcurrant jelly
1 teaspoon (5 ml) wholegrain mustard
$\frac{1}{3}$ pint (200 ml) double cream
salt and pepper

Chop any large mushrooms in half and sauté gently in the butter for two or three minutes. Cool slightly. Combine all the other ingredients in a bowl – use a small whisk to mix in the redcurrant jelly. Season with salt and pepper. Pack the mushrooms into the ramekins and pour over the sauce.

Serve as an *hors d'oeuvre* with chunky bread to soak up the juice. It can be served warm on a cold day.

Promoting health at Cragside

Sir William Armstrong was a hydraulics engineer, a knowledge that he put to good use when he had his fine house built at Cragside in Northumberland. Apart from installing the first electric light system in a private house, he commissioned his architect, Richard Norman Shaw, to build a Turkish Bath and related rooms. Disrobing in the dressing-room, the bather entered the hot-air bath, where water was poured through the grille in the floor on to heated pipes, to produce steam. The bather then had a shower before immersion in the plunge bath.

KEDLESTON DEEP PAN PIZZA

Pizza Base

3 fl oz (75 ml) tepid milk

1 teaspoon (5 ml) sugar

1½ teaspoons (7.5 ml) dried yeast

8 oz (225 g) wholewheat flour

1 teaspoon (5 ml) salt

1 egg, lightly beaten

1 fl oz (30 ml) olive oil

Topping

2 tablespoons (30 ml) olive oil

1 onion, chopped

1 clove of garlic, crushed

2 sticks of celery, finely sliced

¼ pint (150 ml) tomato sauce (use the sauce from Boxhill – Tortellini with Tomato Sauce)

4 oz (125 g) cheese, grated

1 red or green pepper, chopped

1 small tin chickpeas, drained

a few black olives

mixed herbs

2 tablespoons (30 ml) olive oil

Preheat oven: 425°F, 220°C; gas mark 7.

Into a measuring jug pour the tepid milk and whisk in the sugar, sprinkle in the yeast and stir once. Leave on one side for about 10 minutes until it gets a nice frothy head, like a glass of beer. Sift the flour and salt together in a mixing bowl. Then pour in the frothy yeast mixture, beaten egg and olive oil and mix to a firm dough which will leave the sides of the bowl clean. Turn the dough on to a clean work surface and knead for about 10 minutes until the texture becomes smooth and pliable. Put the dough back into the mixing bowl, cover with a piece of cling film and leave until the dough has doubled in size – about 1–1½ hours.

To make the topping gently fry the onion and garlic in oil for 3–4 minutes, add the sliced celery and cook for a further 5 minutes.

Take the dough out of the bowl and 'knock back' to remove any large pockets of air. Knead for a couple of minutes, then press into a well-greased 8 in (20 cm) sandwich tin.

Spread the dough with the tomato sauce, cover with the onions, garlic and celery and with the cheese. Top with the peppers, chickpeas, olives and herbs. Next drizzle the olive oil over everything and bake on a high shelf for about 20–30 minutes until the topping is bubbling and golden and the bread base puffed up. Serve at once with a green salad.

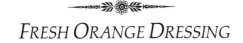

COURGETTE TART

Pastry

4 oz (125 g) plain white flour
pinch salt
1 oz (25 g) butter or margarine

1 oz (25 g) vegetarian lard
cold water

Filling

2 oz (50 g) butter
1 medium onion, chopped
8 oz (225 g) courgettes, sliced
$\frac{1}{2}$ teaspoon (2.5 ml) savory (or other herb of your choice)

2 eggs, lightly beaten
$\frac{1}{4}$ pint (150 ml) creamy milk
2 tablespoons (30 ml) Parmesan cheese, grated

Preheat oven: 350°F, 180°C; gas mark 4.

Sift the flour and salt into a mixing bowl. Cut the fat into small cubes and add to the flour. Using your fingertips, lightly rub the fat into the flour until the mixture looks uniformly crumbly. Sprinkle on 2 tablespoons (30 ml) cold water and draw together with a knife to bring the pastry together, adding a little more water if necessary. Then with your hands, form a smooth ball dough that leaves the sides of the bowl clean. Roll out the pastry and line a greased 7 in (18 cm) flan tin. Prick with a fork and bake for 15 minutes on a preheated baking sheet in the centre of the oven.

For the filling, melt the butter in a saucepan and sweat the onion for a few minutes, add the courgettes and savory and continue to cook until the courgettes are just tender.

Place the onion and courgettes in the pastry case. Mix together the eggs, milk, 1 tablespoon of the Parmesan cheese and salt and pepper and pour over the top. Sprinkle over the remaining Parmesan cheese and bake for 30 minutes.

FRESH ORANGE DRESSING

juice $1\frac{1}{2}$ oranges
1 teaspoon (5 ml) orange rind
1 tablespoon (15 ml) sunflower oil

1 clove of garlic, crushed
salt and pepper

A very simple recipe – just mix together all the ingredients and use with any salad. It would go well with Buckland Abbey Carrot, Raisin and Sesame Seed Salad on p. 32. Makes sufficient to dress a bowl of salad for four.

ONION AND CHEESE SWIRL LOAF

Brown bread dough (use the
Wholemeal Bread recipe from
Erddig on p. 81). Place in a greased
polythene bag to rise instead of in a
loaf tin.

1 oz (25 g) butter
2 small onions, chopped
4 oz (125 g) red Leicester cheese, grated
fresh herbs of your choice
salt and pepper
paprika

Preheat oven: 450°F, 230°C; gas mark 8.

Once the dough has finished 'proving', take out of the polythene bag and roll out on a clean working surface into a rectangle approximately 8 × 14 in (20 × 35.5 cm).

Melt the butter and sweat the chopped onions until transparent. Spread them along the length of the dough piece together with the grated cheese and herbs. Season well with salt and pepper and roll up firmly like a Swiss roll and place on to a greased baking tray. Place the tray inside the polythene bag and once again leave to rise for 30 minutes. Take out of the bag, dust the top with paprika, and bake in a hot oven for 50–60 minutes.

This makes an ideal accompaniment to soup or a salad.

KEDLESTON CARROT CAKE

8 oz (225 g) soft margarine
8 oz (225 g) runny honey
8 oz (225 g) demerara sugar
1 lb (450 g) carrots, grated

1 lb (450 g) plain flour
1 oz (25 g) ground cinnamon
1 oz (25 g) baking powder

Preheat oven: 350°F, 180°C; gas mark 4.

Line an 8 in (20 cm) cake tin. In a large mixing bowl stir together the soft margarine and honey. They will look separated but this does not matter. Add the sugar and carrot and continue to mix. Sieve together all the dry ingredients and stir into the mixture gradually until well and evenly combined.

Spoon into the prepared tin and bake for $1\frac{1}{2}$ hours or until a skewer piercing the cake comes out clean. Turn out on to a wire rack and remove the lining paper.

Don't worry, the eggs have not been forgotten in this recipe – there aren't any!

KINGSTON LACY

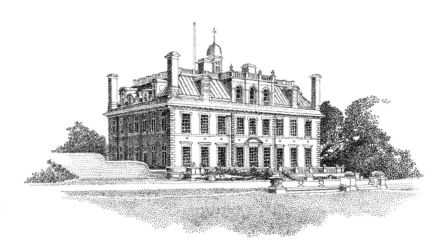

THE lives of the Bankes family have been woven into the fabric of Kingston Lacy since Sir John Bankes, Charles I's Chief Justice, bought the land on which the present house is built, together with Corfe Castle. Fortunes fluctuate: Sir John's wife, brave Dame Mary, whose statue dominates the first flight of the marble staircase at Kingston Lacy, withstood two Civil War sieges at Corfe before the castle was sacked and ruined; her son, Sir Ralph, back in favour, built a new family seat at Kingston Lacy in mellow red brick, the bones of today's house. He also laid the foundation of Kingston Lacy's glory, the magnificent collection of paintings. Kingston Lacy is no soulless gallery, however; the Bankes family loved their house and altered and improved it whilst adding to the Lelys and Van Dycks of Sir Ralph's original collection.

No one did more for Kingston Lacy than William John Bankes, 'the father of all mischiefs' according to his bosom friend, Lord Byron. He and architect Sir Charles Barry transformed Kingston Lacy into the handsome house we see today. They faced it with Chilmark stone, fashioned a new classical entrance hall, a sumptuous marble staircase and loggia as a setting for William's collection of bronzes and marbles, and arranged the state rooms in today's pattern. An enthusiastic traveller and explorer, William sent home a rich variety of treasures, including Sebastian de Piombo's masterpiece *The Judgement of Solomon* which dominates the Dining Room. The great Saloon has pictures banked three deep on every wall, notably two aristocratic Italian beauties by Rubens and a noble Titian. He erected the obelisk of Philae in the grounds, constructed a jewel of a room hung in leather to display his Spanish collection, and bought carvings and furniture.

Banished abroad in disgrace for a sexual indiscretion, he nevertheless continued to commission fittings in wood and marble, shipping them home and writing long letters to his sister on where to put them, until his death in 1855.

Another formidable lady left her mark on the Drawing Room: Henrietta Bankes reigned, first as wife, then during a long widowhood from 1897 and the room is just as she decorated it with rose damask walls, French furniture and a clutter of workboxes, miniatures, plants and ornaments. It was her son, Ralph, who bequeathed the house and all its contents to the Trust, the greatest legacy it has ever received.

Beyond the kitchen courtyard is the red-brick stables where visitors can now have the unusual experience of eating in a private loosebox complete with manger and hay basket, or on a fine day in the pretty flower-filled courtyard. Recipes include unusual salads, good soups, a particularly delicious lasagne and a Chocolate Muesli Bar too good to miss.

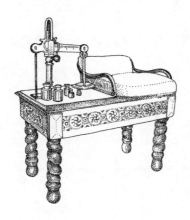

Over-indulgence at Belton

On 29 October 1695, William III visited Sir John Brownlow to admire his newly completed house at Belton in Lincolnshire. According to the diarist De La Pryme, the King was 'mighty nobly entertained.... Sir John killed twelve fat oxen and 60 sheep besides other victuals for his entertainment ... The King was exceeding merry and drank freely which was the occasion that when he came to Lincoln he could eat nothing but a mess of milk.'

The cookery and household books belonging to Henrietta Bankes are preserved at Kingston Lacy. Henrietta was the wife of Walter Ralph Bankes, and came to Kingston Lacy after her marriage in 1897. Here is her recipe for 'anyone overworked or below par':

2 oz (50 g) salsaperella	$\frac{1}{2}$ pt (250 ml) black beer
2 oz (50 g) peruvian bark	$\frac{3}{4}$ pt (400 ml) old rum
$\frac{1}{2}$ oz (12 g) gentian root	2 pt (1.25 l) cold water
$\frac{1}{2}$ lb (225 g) sugar candy	1 pt (500 ml) hot water

Place 2 pt (1.25 l) cold water with the herbs on the oven all night. Strain off the liquid next morning, then rinse with 1 pt (500 ml) boiling water, and after again straining, boil both the pints and the quarts of water with the sugar candy until the candy is dissolved. When cold, add the black beer and rum. 1 wineglass in a morning and evening if required.

TOMATO AND CHEESE SOUP

2 medium onions, finely chopped	1 dessertspoon (10 ml) red wine vinegar
2 oz (50 g) butter	1 pint (500 ml) milk
1 oz (25 g) flour	salt and pepper
6 oz (175 g) tomato purée	3 oz (75 g) Cheddar cheese, grated
1 pint (500 ml) vegetable stock	parsley, chopped

In a large saucepan, sauté the finely chopped onions in butter until soft. Stir in the flour and cook for a minute or two before adding the tomato purée, vegetable stock and red wine vinegar. Bring to the boil, stirring all the time and simmer for 5–10 minutes. Take off the heat and blend in a food processor (alternatively, it tastes just as good left as it is). Return to the pan, pour in the milk and season with salt and pepper. Reheat the soup, but don't let it boil, and stir in half the grated Cheddar cheese. Ladle into individual bowls and top with the remainder of the grated cheese and finely chopped parsley mixed together.

Economical and fast, yet with a subtle tangy flavour – a useful recipe as it consists of only staples from the store cupboard.

CURRIED BROWN RICE SALAD

6 oz (175 g) brown rice
2 oz (50 g) coarsely chopped walnuts
2 oz (50 g) raisins
2 eating apples, chopped

1 tablespoon (15 ml) curry powder
combined with 6 tablespoons
(90 ml) French dressing
1 tablespoon (15 ml) parsley, freshly
chopped

Cook the rice as described on the packet, drain and allow to cool slightly. In a salad bowl combine the walnuts, raisins, chopped apple and curry dressing. When the rice is lukewarm, tip it into the bowl and gently mix with the other ingredients with a wooden spoon. Lastly sprinkle on the chopped parsley for added colour.

A nutty, spicy salad.

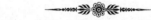

MUSHROOM AND TARRAGON SALAD

1 lb (450 g) mushrooms
1 dessertspoon (10 ml) dried tarragon
(or fresh if you have it)

8 tablespoons (120 ml) vinaigrette
dressing
salt and pepper

Wipe the mushrooms if necessary and slice. Gently mix in the tarragon, vinaigrette dressing and salt and pepper.

Good too, made with fresh mint if tarragon isn't available.

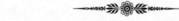

CARROT AND COCONUT SALAD

1 lb (450 g) carrots
3 tablespoons (45 ml) dessicated coconut
$\frac{1}{2}$ teaspoon (2.5 ml) ground ginger
2 oz (50 g) sultanas

4 tablespoons (60 ml) vinaigrette
dressing
salt and freshly ground black pepper

Peel and coarsely grate the carrots. Mix all the other ingredients together and season with salt and pepper.

Economical and exotic!

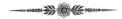

VEGETARIAN LASAGNE

Vegetable Sauce

2 oz (50 g) butter
1 onion, finely chopped
1 clove of garlic, crushed
1 red or green pepper, diced
12 oz (350 g) mixed vegetables, chopped
 (courgettes, carrots, French beans,
 peas, broad beans)

4 oz (125 g) tinned or frozen sweetcorn
1 small tin tomatoes
2 tablespoons (30 ml) tomato purée
1 teaspoon (2.5 ml) dried oregano
4 oz (125 g) tinned, drained kidney
 beans
salt and pepper

Béchamel Sauce

$1\frac{1}{2}$ oz (37 g) butter
$1\frac{1}{2}$ oz (37 g) flour
$\frac{3}{4}$ pint (400 ml) milk

grated nutmeg
salt and pepper

Topping

4 oz (125 g) Parmesan and Cheddar
 cheese, grated, mixed to dust on the
 lasagne layers

Lasagne

12 oz (350 g) oven-ready or pre-cooked
 lasagne

Preheat oven: 375°F, 190°C; gas mark 5.

Melt the butter in a large saucepan and fry the onion for 10 minutes until soft but not browned. Add the garlic, diced pepper and the chopped vegetables and continue to fry for a few minutes, stirring now and then before mixing in the sweetcorn, tinned tomatoes, tomato purée and the oregano. Place a lid on the pan and simmer for 20 minutes or until the vegetables are tender. Take off the heat, stir in the drained kidney beans and season with salt and pepper.

To make the sauce, melt the butter in a saucepan, stir in the flour and cook for a minute or two before pouring in the milk. Stirring all the time, bring to the boil, then add the nutmeg, salt and pepper.

Have the pasta and sauce all ready. Put a layer of the vegetable sauce on the bottom of an ovenproof dish. Cover with a thin layer of béchamel sauce, dust with cheese and place a layer of lasagne sheets on top. Continue like this until all the ingredients are used up, ending with the béchamel sauce, sprinkled with cheese.

Bake in the oven for 30–40 minutes until the top is golden.

CHOCOLATE MUESLI BAR

3 oz (75 g) butter
1 tablespoon (15 ml) golden syrup
8 oz (225 g) muesli
2 oz (50 g) dates, chopped

2 oz (50 g) dried apricots, chopped
2 oz (50 g) walnuts and almonds,
  chopped
4 oz (125 g) plain chocolate

Melt the butter and golden syrup in a saucepan. Remove from the heat and add all the ingredients except the chocolate. Press into a rectangular or square tin and allow to set. Very gently melt the chocolate and spread over the biscuit mixture. Allow to set once again, then cut into fingers.

DORSET APPLE CAKE

8 oz (225 g) eating apples
4 oz (125 g) butter
4 oz (125 g) demerara sugar
8 oz (225 g) self-raising flour

1 teaspoon (5 ml) ground cinnamon
2 eggs, lightly beaten
icing sugar

Preheat oven: 350°F, 180°C; gas mark 4.

Grease and line an 8 in (20 cm) cake tin. Peel, core and roughly chop the apples. In a mixing bowl, cream together the butter and sugar until light and fluffy. Sieve the flour and cinnamon and add alternately with the eggs into the sugar and butter; adding these ingredients alternately stops the eggs curdling. Stir in the chopped apple and spoon into the prepared tin.

Bake in the oven for 50 minutes. Cool slightly before turning out on to a wire rack to cool. When cold, dust the top with icing sugar. Good served warm as a pudding with some clotted cream.

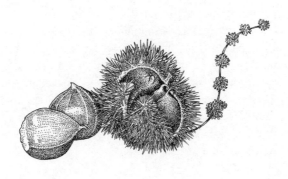

MONTACUTE HOUSE

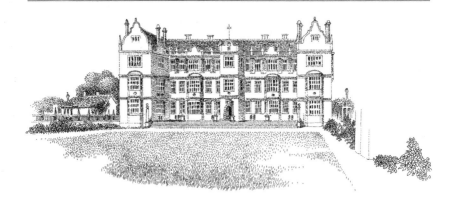

Montacute is a golden Elizabethan house, a wonderful amalgam of Gothic and Renaissance. Sir Edward Phelips, a successful lawyer, built the house in the last years of the sixteenth century with the help of a Somerset mason, William Arnold. Arnold was able to introduce the latest Renaissance detail – shell-headed niches, obelisks and a symmetrical plan – yet the house remains firmly embedded in the Gothic, with reminders of chivalric pageantry, romantic evocations beloved by the Elizabethans.

Beyond the outbuildings and kitchen gardens lies the village of Montacute, with the sharp hill, *mons acutus,* that gives the village and the house their name. Beyond the formal gardens and tree-lined avenues is the green countryside of Somerset, sheep and somnolent cows grazing peacefully in a quintessentially English landscape.

The Phelips family lived there for three centuries. As their fortunes waxed and waned, so did Montacute's, sometimes richly furnished and sometimes neglected. Wills of byzantine complexity and family squabbles decimated the Phelips' inheritance, so that by the twentieth century the estate was insolvent. After years of letting, the house was in such poor repair that in 1931 it was valued for £5,882 'for scrap' and in grave danger of demolition. Montacute was rescued and given to the Trust, but the problem of furnishing the house remained. Generous individuals and organisations have lent or given furniture, pictures and furnishings so that the rooms are now furnished in appropriately spare fashion. Phelips portraits from every century watch today's visitors admiring the impressive stone screen in the hall, the intriguing plasterwork and the massive Ham stone fireplaces. Lord Curzon, a famous tenant, is remembered by a bedroom containing a huge bath in a Jacobean-style cupboard, the nearest to twentieth-century convenience to be found in this very traditional house.

Climb the stairs to the second floor to find the largest long gallery to survive in England: 172 feet long with oriel windows at each end giving wonderful views of garden and countryside. The National Portrait Gallery has hung here a fascinating collection of Tudor and Jacobean portraits. Beautiful and ugly, noble and not so noble, happy and sad, the faces bring to life those who influenced this turbulent period of English history.

In bad weather, the Elizabethans used the Long Gallery for gentle exercise. When fine, they strolled the walled gardens as we do today, admiring the grand façades of the great house, the beautifully clipped hedges and well-kept beds. Behind a huge yew hedge planted to allow servants to reach the kitchen gardens (now the car parks) unobserved, you will find the old laundry and bakehouse, now the restaurant. Old mullioned windows, low ceilings and pink lacy tablecloths provide a homely background to carefully cooked, imaginative recipes. Local ingredients feature largely. In Golden Cider Soup, local cider is an essential ingredient which produces one of the best soups I have ever tasted.

While the Phelips family were enjoying a good diet in their great house at Montacute, with plenty of fresh fruit and vegetables produced by the extensive kitchen garden, their tenants in the adjacent village were faring less well. An extract from *The Skeleton at the Plough, 1827–46*, an autobiographical account by George Mitchell, gives some idea of their daily diet:

Our food consisted principally of a little barley-cake, potatoes, salt, tea kettle broth and barley 'flippet'. Tea kettle broth consisted of a few pieces of bread soaked in hot water with a little salt, sometimes with a leek chopped up in it. Never had I ever a sufficient quantity of bread being used for the spoon to stand upright in. Barley flippet was made by sprinkling barley-meal into a pot of boiling water which when sufficiently thickened was served up with salt and a little treacle.

Sometimes, I would pull a turnip from the field and gnaw it to prevent hunger ... If I could find peas, beans or carrots, I would eat as many as I could get and many a time have I hunted and foraged about for snails in the hedges and roasted them for my lunch and tea.

From an exhibition mounted by the Montacute Parish Council in one of the garden pavilions at Montacute.

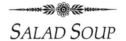

GOLDEN CIDER SOUP

2 oz (50 g) butter	14 oz (400 g) tin chopped tomatoes
8 oz (225 g) carrots, diced	$\frac{3}{4}$ pt (400 ml) medium or sweet cider
8 oz (225 g) potatoes, diced	$\frac{3}{4}$ pt (400 ml) vegetable stock
2 cloves of garlic, crushed	salt and freshly ground pepper

Melt the butter in a large saucepan and sweat the diced carrots and potatoes for 5 minutes. Add the crushed garlic, tin of tomatoes, cider and vegetable stock and bring to the boil. Cover and simmer until the vegetables are tender. Season with salt and pepper. Pour into a food processor and blend until very smooth. Return to the pan and reheat before serving.

The cider gives this simple recipe a wonderful, luxurious flavour.

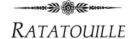

SALAD SOUP

1 onion, finely chopped	4 radishes, chopped
2 oz (50 g) butter	4 tomatoes, quartered
1 lettuce, shredded	2 punnets of mustard and cress
1 green pepper, diced	vegetable stock
$\frac{1}{2}$ cucumber, peeled and diced	salt and pepper

In a large saucepan sauté the chopped onion in the butter until soft. Add the shredded lettuce, diced green pepper, peeled and diced cucumber, chopped radishes, quartered tomatoes and most of the mustard and cress. Add sufficient vegetable stock to cover. Simmer until everything is soft, then blend in a food processor. Return to the saucepan to reheat before serving. Sprinkle the remainder of the mustard and cress as a garnish to each bowl.

An odd, distinctive flavour – a good soup if the weather turns suddenly cold in high summer.

RATATOUILLE

1 onion, coarsely chopped	4 tablespoons (60 ml) olive oil
2 cloves of garlic, crushed	14 oz (400 g) tin tomatoes
1 small aubergine, diced into chunks	1 teaspoon (5 ml) mixed herbs
2 courgettes, sliced	salt and freshly ground black pepper
4 oz (125 g) mushrooms, sliced	

In a large saucepan sauté the prepared vegetables in olive oil until they are beginning to soften. Add the tin of tomatoes and herbs, bring to the boil and then put a lid on the saucepan. Turn down the heat and leave to cook gently for 40 minutes. Season with salt and pepper before serving.

Use this recipe as a vegetable accompaniment or to stuff the pancakes from Berrington Hall on p. 16.

Ratatouille Soup

Cool the above ratatouille mixture and blend in a food processor. Return to the saucepan and stir in $1\frac{1}{4}$ pints (675 ml) vegetable stock. Reheat and serve piping hot, garnished with parsley.

A truly Mediterranean flavour.

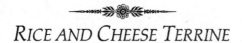

RICE AND CHEESE TERRINE

8 oz (225 g) rice	4–6 oz (125–175 g) cheese, grated
2 oz (50 g) butter	2 tomatoes, chopped
1 onion, chopped	2 eggs, lightly beaten
2 cloves of garlic, crushed	salt and pepper
4 oz (125 g) mixed vegetables, diced	6 oz (175 g) red peppers, chopped
(you can use frozen if in a hurry)	

Preheat oven: 350°F, 180°C; gas mark 4.

Cook the rice, preferably in some vegetable stock, until tender. Melt the butter in a saucepan and sweat the onion and garlic until transparent. Cook the vegetables of your choice. In a mixing bowl combine all the ingredients, except the red peppers, and season well.

Line a 2 lb (900 g) loaf tin with non-stick paper. Layer half the rice mixture into the tin, spread over the chopped red peppers and add a final layer of the balance of the mixture. Cover with foil and bake in the oven for 1 hour. Cool slightly before turning out carefully and removing the lining paper.

Serve hot or cold. If serving hot, the Mushroom and Wine Sauce from Kedleston (p. 85) or the Tomato Sauce from Box Hill (p. 21) would go well with the terrine.

SOMERSET QUICHE

Pastry

3 oz (75 g) Cheddar cheese, grated
6 oz (175 g) plain flour
pinch of mustard
salt and pepper

3 oz (75 g) butter or margarine
1 egg yolk
cold water

Filling

1 large onion, chopped
2 oz (50 g) butter
4 oz (125 g) fresh white bread-crumbs
½ pt (250 ml) milk
2 bay leaves

3 eggs
2 oz (50 g) clotted cream (or extra
    double cream if clotted
    unobtainable)
salt and pepper

Preheat oven: 400°F, 200°C; gas mark 6.

Grate the cheddar cheese. In a large mixing bowl place the flour, mustard and seasoning. Cut the fat into small cubes and rub into the flour, using your fingertips until the mixture resembles fine bread-crumbs. Tip in the grated cheese and combine well. Add the egg yolk and one tablespoon (15 ml) of cold water and draw together with a knife and then your fingers to form a dough (if necessary add a little more water). Knead slightly, then, ideally, chill in a polythene bag in the fridge for around 30 minutes.

Put a baking sheet into the centre of the oven to heat up. Roll out the pastry and line a greased 9 in (23 cm) tin. Prick the base all over, place on the baking sheet and bake for 15 minutes or until the pastry is firm.

Turn the oven down to 350°F, 180°C, gas mark 4. Sweat the chopped onion in the butter and place in the pastry case with the bread-crumbs. In a small saucepan infuse the milk with the bay leaves. Remove from the heat and pour over the bread-crumbs. Whisk together the eggs, clotted cream and seasoning and pour into the flan case. Place on the baking sheet and bake for 35–40 minutes or until the filling is set and lightly browned.

Fresh bay leaves are essential for the flavour.

STILTON AND WALNUT QUICHE

10 oz (300 g) wholewheat pastry (use
    the recipe from Chirk, Country
    Cheese Tart p. 61)
6 oz (175 g) crumbled Stilton cheese

4 oz (125 g) chopped walnuts
3 eggs
½ pt (250 ml) milk
salt and pepper

Preheat oven: 350°F, 180°C; gas mark 4. (Place a baking sheet in the centre.)

Prepare the pastry case as previously described.

Sprinkle the crumbled Stilton and chopped walnuts on the base of the case. Whisk together the eggs and milk and season well. Pour carefully into the flan and place in the centre of oven on the baking sheet. Bake for 40–45 minutes. Leave to cool for around 10–15 minutes to allow the filling to 'firm up' before serving.

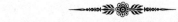

JOE'S PICKLE

1 lb (450 g) onions, peeled
1½ (675 g) cooking apples, peeled and cored
1 lb (450 g) stoned dates
1 lb (450 g) sultanas

1 lb (450 g) soft brown sugar
1 level teaspoon (4 ml) salt
pinch of cayenne
scant 1 pt (500 ml) spiced or pickling vinegar

Coarsely chop the onions, apples and dates in a food processor (make sure you leave some texture) and place in a large mixing bowl. Add in the sultanas, sugar, salt and cayenne and pour on the vinegar. Mix well. Cover with a cloth overnight (add extra vinegar if necessary), pack into jars and cover with a waxed disc and cellophane. This will keep for around 6 months.

At Montacute it is served with Somerset Cheddar as a Ploughman's Lunch, but it also makes a good present for pickle lovers.

RHUBARB AND ORANGE TART

Pastry

4 oz (125 g) plain flour sifted with ½ teaspoon (2.5 ml) cinammon and a pinch of salt
3 oz (75 g) butter

1 oz (25 g) caster sugar
1 egg yolk
1 tablespoon (15 ml) cold water

Filling

1½ lb (675 g) rhubarb
3 oz (75 g) dark brown sugar

juice and rind of 1 orange

Topping

2 egg whites, beaten

4 oz (125 g) caster sugar

Preheat oven: 400°F, 200°C; gas mark 6.

Use the pastry instructions as for Lemon Tart from Chirk (p. 62) and bake blind in an 8 in (20 cm) flan tin for 15–20 minutes.

To make the filling, cut the rhubarb into manageable lengths and place in a saucepan with the sugar and juice and rind of an orange. Heat gently and cook until barely tender (test for sweetness – you may need to add a little more sugar). Place in the pre-baked pastry case.

For the topping, beat together two egg whites until stiff and fold in 4 oz (125 g) caster sugar. Pile this on the pudding and bake for 15–20 minutes until pale brown and set. Serve hot or cold.

SOMERSET CIDER CAKE

8 oz (225 g) sultanas	2 eggs
$\frac{1}{4}$ pt (150 ml) sweet or medium dry cider	8 oz (225 g) plain flour
4 oz (125 g) butter	1 teaspoon (5 ml) bicarbonate of soda
4 oz (125 g) soft light brown sugar	

Topping

3 oz (75 g) butter	1 teaspoon (5 ml) lemon juice
6 oz (175 g) icing sugar	1 tablespoon (15 ml) runny honey

Preheat oven: 350°F, 180°C; gas mark 4.

Grease and line an 8 in (20 cm) cake tin.

Soak the sultanas overnight in the cider. Cream together the butter and sugar until light and fluffy. Gradually beat in the eggs one at a time. Fold in half the flour and the bicarbonate of soda, then the sultanas and cider and lastly the balance of the flour.

Bake in the centre of the oven for approximately 1 hour or until a skewer comes out clean. Cool slightly before turning out on to a wire rack and remove the lining paper.

For the topping, whisk the butter until light. Add the balance of the ingredients and continue whisking until well combined. When the cake is completely cold, spoon on the topping and fork over until it looks like a candlewick bath mat!

MOSELEY OLD HALL

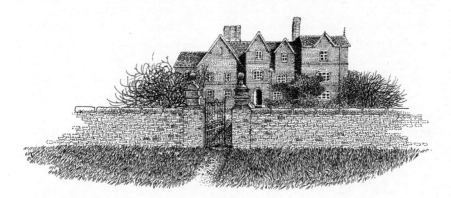

MOSELEY OLD HALL in Staffordshire is cared for by the National Trust because it has a special association with a particular person and period in English history.

From the outside, Moseley appears a small, nineteenth-century red-brick house; no clue here to its significance, though an expert on garden design might pause over the elaborate seventeenth-century knot garden.

But step through the heavily studded back door and you are in a timber-framed house of the middle years of the seventeenth century; more specifically the morning of 8 September 1651, when this modest house and its worthy, but not aristocratic, family, the Whitgreaves, were swept up in the bloody civil war then raging between Royalists and Parliamentarians. Charles I had been executed two years earlier, but his eldest son, later Charles II, had met in battle Cromwell's forces at Worcester on 3 September and had been heavily defeated. On the run with £1,000 (a huge figure in those days) on his head, Charles finally reached Moseley. Thomas Whitgreave, 'The Preserver', and his mother, Dame Alice, were Catholics and Royalist sympathisers; they sheltered the desperate man for two days until his escape to Bristol and later to France, disguised as serving man to Jane Lane, a near neighbour. You can see the heartfelt letter of thanks he wrote Jane in the hall at Moseley.

Thomas wrote a detailed account of those two days, and, retracing Charles's steps through the house, the events still seem vivid. The house is furnished just as it would have been in 1651. In the bedroom is the heavy oak four-poster bed in which the exhausted man slept; through a door you can see the small hiding place into which tall Charles – he was over 6 foot – crammed his body when soldiers came to search the grounds and to interrogate Thomas. From the small windows above the porch he watched with Thomas and the local priest, Father John Huddlestone, the bedraggled

103

remnants of his army making their slow way north back to Scotland. Under the eaves is the little oratory, a tranquil evocative room. Perhaps Charles experienced some spiritual solace here, for he called it 'a very decent place' and years later, when he was dying, summoned Father Huddlestone who received him into the Catholic faith and administered the last rites.

Portraits and mementoes bring alive those momentous events, and local schools today spend whole days at Moseley making seventeenth-century recipes and rush lights, and experiencing for themselves that earlier world. Outside, a seventeenth-century garden has been recreated, old herbaceous plants, shrubs and roses filling the beds; there is a formal knot garden and old varieties of fruit – quinces, mulberries and medlars – flourish.

Beyond the back garden is a barn; upstairs is the restaurant. Tea menus include traditional tarts using fruits from the garden, and from time to time there are special candle-lit suppers and lunches featuring old recipes such as Dame Alice Soup.

———◦◦◦◦◦⫸⟫ ❀ ⟪⫷◦◦◦◦◦———

DAME ALICE SOUP

1 small onion, chopped

2 small carrots, chopped

2 oz (50 g) butter

1 bayleaf

1 teaspoon (5 ml) celery seeds (these are essential)

1 teaspoon (5 ml) fresh thyme

1 teaspoon (5 ml) fresh parsley

6 peppercorns

2 oz (50 g) plain flour

$1\frac{1}{4}$ pt (675 ml) vegetable stock

$\frac{1}{2}$ pt (250 ml) milk

salt and pepper

1 teaspoon (5 ml) Marmite

Fry the chopped onion and carrots in the butter in a large saucepan for a minute or two. Add the bayleaf, celery seeds, thyme, parsley and peppercorns, and continue to cook to bring out the flavours of the herbs. Stir in the flour, add the stock and bring to the boil, stirring frequently. Simmer gently for 15 minutes. Pour in the milk, season with salt and pepper and stir in the Marmite. Bring almost to the boil and servce.

This is based on a very old recipe. Dame Alice Whitgreave was the mother of Thomas 'The Preserver' and helped to shelter Charles II in 1651.

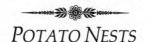

ALMONDINES

2 lb (900 g) potatoes	1 dessertspoon (10 ml) fresh chopped
1 oz (25 g) butter	herbs
3 tablespoons (45 ml) ground almonds	salt and pepper
1 egg	4–6 oz (125–175 g) flaked almonds

Preheat oven: 375°F, 190°C; gas mark 5.

Peel the potatoes and chop them roughly. Cook them in salted water until tender, drain and mash with the butter. Add the egg, herbs and salt and pepper to taste. Form into small balls, about the size of small plums, and roll in the flaked almonds. Chill for about 30 minutes in the fridge.

Place the almond balls on a lightly greased baking sheet and bake in the preheated oven for 15–20 minutes until they are lightly golden.

POTATO NESTS

Make up the same potato mixture as for 'Almondines' above.

Filling

8 oz (225 g) carrots, roughly chopped	1 oz (25 g) butter
1 clove of garlic, unpeeled	salt and pepper

Preheat oven: 350°F, 180°C; gas mark 4.

Pipe the potato mixture into nest shapes, $2\frac{1}{2}$ in (6.25 cm) across, on a greased baking sheet and bake in the oven for 15 minutes.

Boil the carrots with the unpeeled garlic until cooked. Drain and pop the garlic out of its skin. Blend the carrots and garlic in a food processor with the butter until you have a purée. Season with salt and pepper. Put a spoonful of purée into each nest and put back in the oven for a further 10–15 minutes.

Alternative Fillings

Fresh tomato sauce – see Box Hill Tortellini with Tomato Sauce, p. 21.
Spinach mixture – see Charlecote Pinenut and Spinach Jalousie, p. 53.

SPINACH TART WITH THREE CHEESES

12 oz (350 g) wholemeal pastry (use the
*   pastry recipe for Brownsea Celery,*
*   Apple and Mushroom Quiche on*
*   p. 25)*

Filling

1 medium onion, finely chopped
1 clove of garlic, crushed
1 oz (25 g) butter
1 lb (450 g) frozen spinach
2 eggs, lightly beaten

2 tablespoons (30 ml) Parmesan cheese
8 oz (225 g) curd cheese
4 oz (125 g) Mozzarella cheese cut into
*   little cubes*

Preheat oven: 350°F, 180°C; gas mark 4.

Make up the pastry as previously instructed and reserve a third. Prepare and bake the pastry case in a 9 in (23 cm) tin on a baking sheet in the centre of the oven.

Sweat the onion and garlic with the butter until soft. Defrost, cook and drain well the spinach – cool slightly and stir in the onion and garlic together with the lightly beaten eggs. Add the three cheeses, season with salt and pepper and spoon into the pastry case.

Roll out the balance of the pastry and cut strips long enough to make a criss-cross pattern all over the surface of the tart. Brush the strips with milk and place the tart on the baking sheet in the oven. Bake for about 30–40 minutes.

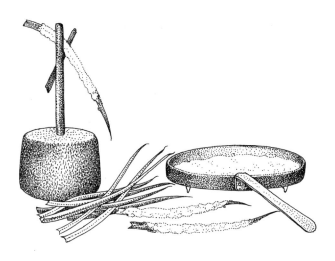

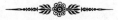

MULBERRY AND APPLE PLATE PIE

Shortcrust Pastry

8 oz (225 g) plain flour
2 oz (50 g) vegetarian lard
2 oz (50 g) butter

pinch of salt
cold water to mix

Filling

1 lb (450 g) cooking apples
8 oz (225 g) mulberries

3 oz (75 g) sugar
2 tablespoons (30 ml) water

Preheat oven: 400°F, 200°C, gas mark 6.

Make up the pastry in the same method as Chirk Country Cheese Tart (p. 61) and leave to rest.

Peel and slice the apples thinly into a saucepan together with the mulberries. Mix in the sugar and water and cook gently for about 10 minutes until the fruit is soft. Adjust the sweetness if necessary. Leave to cool.

Preheat the oven, put in a baking sheet and lightly grease a 10 in (25 cm) pie plate. Roll out a little more than half the pastry and line the plate, pressing it gently and firmly. Spoon in the cooled filling, then roll out the other half of the pastry to form a lid. Brush the bottom layer of pastry round the edge with water, then fix the pastry lid into place. Trim the edges and use any trimmings as decoration. Make a hole in the centre for the steam. Brush with milk and sprinkle on a dusting of caster sugar.

Place the pie on a baking sheet and bake for 30 minutes.

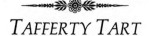

TAFFERTY TART

12 oz (350 g) shortcrust pastry (using the amounts and method for Moseley Mulberry and Apple Pie, above)
8 large cooking apples, thinly sliced

5 oz (150 g) sugar blended with the grated rind of 1 lemon and some of the lemon pulp, finely chopped
butter

Topping

4–6 oz (125–175 g) icing sugar
1 tablespoon (15 ml) milk

1 tablespoon (15 ml) lemon juice

Preheat oven: 400°F, 200°C; gas mark 6.

Grease a 10 in (25 cm) pie plate. Roll out over half of the pastry and line the plate, pressing it gently and firmly into place. Arrange the thinly sliced apples in layers, sprinkling each layer with the lemon and sugar mixture. Dot with butter and cover with the remainder of the pastry arranged in lattice strips. Place in the oven on a baking sheet and bake for 35 minutes.

While warm, drizzle with the topping made by mixing the ingredients together to produce a pouring consistency.

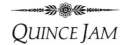

QUINCE JAM

2 lb (900 g) prepared quinces   juice of 1 lemon
3 lb (1.4kg) sugar   water

Peel, core and chop the quinces into small pieces. Put them in a saucepan with enough water to cover and cook slowly until the fruit is really soft – this takes 20–30 minutes. Then add the sugar and lemon juice and stir until dissolved. Boil rapidly until setting point is reached. Pot and cover in the usual way. Makes about 5 lb (2.3kg).

Quinces ripen in October – when the leaves start to fall – and are even better if used after a frost.

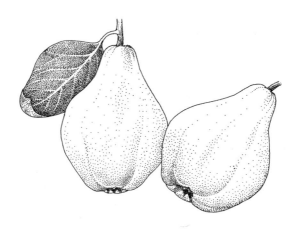

PETWORTH HOUSE

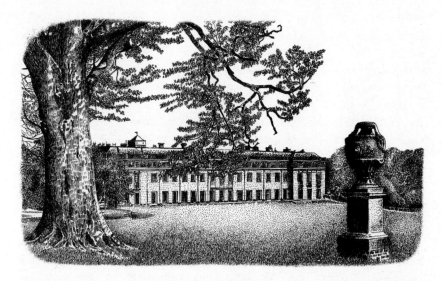

PETWORTH HOUSE is a jewel of a house in a setting as important as itself – Capability Brown's masterpiece. The great west front of the mansion, over 300 foot long, faces 700 acres of park and pleasure gardens with serpentine lakes, islands, temples, folly, rare trees and shrubs, producing a feeling of spaciousness and serenity rare in the crowded south east. Deer graze beneath Brown's carefully placed clumps of trees, in the summer the park hosts picnics and impromptu cricket matches, on the horizon is a turreted Gothick folly, and in the winter – for the park is open all year – the fine views and clean air off the South Downs are enjoyed by both visitors from afar and locals from the town.

This is peculiarly appropriate, since unusually for a 'country house' the cottages, shops and parish church of Petworth huddle right up against the east side of the house, home of the Percy and Wyndham families since 1150. The mansion is a treasure house of paintings, sculpture and carving, collected by the cultured earls of Northumberland and Egremont. The 9th Earl of Northumberland built up a fine library of books, many still at Petworth. After spending sixteen years in the Tower under suspicion of complicity in the Gunpowder Plot, he retired to Petworth to experiment in science and alchemy, earning the nickname of the 'Wizard Earl'. The 6th Duke of Somerset rebuilt the house in 1688, as we see it today, and the 2nd Earl of Egremont collected many of the old masters and antique statuary. Under the benign and humane influence of the 3rd Earl, who held the title for 65 years, Petworth enjoyed its 'golden age'. His hospitality was famous, 'the very animals at Petworth seemed happier than in any other spot on earth'. A great patron of all the arts, he numbered many writers and painters among his friends. Turner spent many years there painting glowing landscapes, many of which still hang in the North Gallery and the Turner Room. The Earl's consuming interest in agriculture led to the promotion of new methods to improve the lot of his tenants – a delightful picture in the North Gallery depicts a feast given by him at Petworth to cheer his workers during a year of depression.

The North Gallery was his creation: on its terracotta-coloured walls are hung works by Turner, Gainsborough, Reynolds, Wilson and Romney and a host of less well-known painters. The 3rd Earl also formed the Carved Room in which cherubs, musical instruments, baskets of flowers, fruit, birds, palm trees, lobsters, crabs, sole and partridges, exquisitely carved in limewood by Grinling Gibbons, John Selden and Jonathan Ritson, tumble from floor to ceiling. Beyond the Carved Room is the Marble Hall and the Beauty Room, so-called because portraits of Queen Anne and all her ladies-in-waiting line the walls.

Cross the lawn at the back of the house and you are in the Stables, now housing a fascinating Archive Room and the great Audit Room where farmers came to pay their dues. It is now the tea-room. Do take tea if you can – Mrs Matthews' cakes are famous and not to be missed. For lunch you will find simple fare, carefully cooked: home-made soup, vegetable bakes served in individual pots and a rich vegetable quiche flavoured with horseradish and herbs.

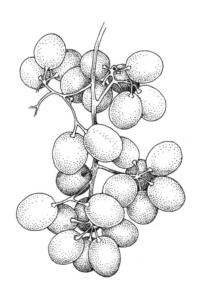

Hospitality and Horticulture at Petworth

George, 3rd Earl of Egremont, was one of the most admired and popular of Petworth's owners. His birthday became an occasion for entertainment of the local populace, and a detailed account of a postponed feast in May 1834 has survived, testifying to his philanthropy:

a fine sight it was; fifty-four tables, each fifty feet long, were placed in a vast semicircle on the lawn before the house. ... two great tents were erected in the middle to receive the provisions, which were conveyed in carts, like ammunition. Plum puddings and loaves were piled like canon-balls, and innumerable joints of boiled and roast beef were spread out, while hot joints were prepared in the kitchen, and sent forth as soon as the firing of guns announced the hour of the feast. Tickets were given to the inhabitants of a certain district, and the number was about 4000; but, as many more came, the Old Peer could not endure that there should be anybody hungering outside the gates, and he went out himself and ordered the barriers to be taken down and admittance given to all. They think 6000 were fed... Nothing could exceed the pleasure of that fine old fellow; he was in and out of the windows of his room twenty times, enjoying the sight of these poor wretches, all attired in their best, cramming themselves and their brats with as much as they could devour, and snatching a day of relaxation and happiness.

The 3rd Earl was keenly interested in agriculture and was amongst the first in England to grow rhubarb.

His grandson, Henry, 1st Lord Leconfield, is said to have spent £3,000 on a banana after a guest had boasted that bananas eaten straight off the tree tasted much better than ones shipped half way round the world. Next morning the head gardener was dispatched to Kew to learn how to grow a banana and told to come back and grow one. A special greenhouse was built and the tree flourished. The day came to sample the results, and the household assembled in silence to witness the event. Using a golden fork, Lord Leconfield tasted the fruit. Furious, he hurled cutlery, plate and banana on to the floor, thundering 'Oh God, it tastes just like any other damn banana!'

VEGETARIAN QUICHE IN WHOLEMEAL HERB PASTRY

Pastry

8 oz (225 g) plain wholemeal flour
1 dessertspoon (10 ml) mixed herbs
pinch of salt

4 oz (125 g) hard margarine
cold water to mix

Filling

1 dessertspoon (10 ml) sunflower oil
1 small onion, sliced
2 tomatoes, sliced
$\frac{1}{2}$ red pepper, sliced
$\frac{1}{2}$ green pepper, sliced
4 oz (125 g) mushrooms, sliced
2 courgettes, sliced
2 sticks of celery, sliced
or use any combination of these
vegetables sufficient to fill the case

1 dessertspoon (10 ml) creamed
horseradish
1 dessertspoon (10 ml) fresh basil
4 eggs
$\frac{1}{4}$ pint (150 ml) milk
$\frac{1}{4}$ pint (150 ml) cream
salt, pepper and Worcestershire sauce
to taste

Topping

a handful of chopped hazelnuts and/or
poppyseeds

Preheat oven: 375°F, 190°C; gas mark 5.

Place flour, herbs and salt in bowl, rub in margarine with fingertips until the consistency of crunchy breadcrumbs and mix with enough water to form a stiff dough. Roll out on a floured board. Line a greased, fluted quiche dish and brush with beaten egg on base and sides to give a crisp pastry.

To make the filling, cook sliced onion in vegetable oil and two teaspoons of water until soft but not brown. Add sliced tomatoes, red and green peppers, sliced mushrooms, courgettes and celery. Cook for 5 minutes stirring often. Add the dessertspoon of horseradish sauce and the dessert-spoon of basil. Stir and cook for a few minutes until thick and creamy.

Beat four eggs into the milk and cream and add salt and pepper and a dash of Worcestershire sauce. Combine the cooked vegetables and egg mixture and pour into pastry case. Chop a handful of hazelnuts and sprinkle on top. Also lightly sprinkle with poppyseed.

Place on a baking tray (most important to ensure that the bottom of pastry is properly cooked) in the middle of a preheated oven and cook for about 40 minutes.

PETWORTH VEGETABLE BAKES

1 cauliflower
1½ lb (675 g) courgettes
1½ oz (37 g) butter
1½ oz (37 g) flour

¾ pt (400 ml) milk
1 teaspoon (5 ml) Dijon mustard
1 teaspoon (5 ml) mixed herbs

Toppings

Either: 1 lb (450 g) cooked, sliced new potatoes and a little melted butter

or: 1 lb (450 g) swede, cooked and mashed until fluffy with butter, salt and lots of freshly ground black pepper

Preheat oven: 325°F, 160°C; gas mark 3.

Divide the cauliflower into florets and slice courgettes into ¼ inch (6 mm) slices. Divide between the four dishes. Make a white sauce: melt the butter in a saucepan, stir in the flour and cook for a minute or two before pouring in the milk. Stirring all the time, bring to the boil, then add a teaspoon of Dijon mustard and one of mixed herbs. Pour over the dishes the white sauce, cover with either of the toppings and cook in the preheated oven for 20 minutes.

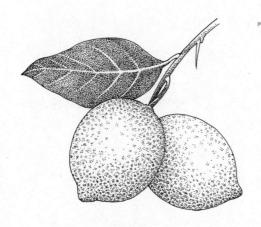

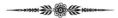

ALMOND TOPPED APRICOT CAKE

Cake

6 oz (175 g) butter, softened

6 oz (175 g) caster sugar

3 eggs

6 oz (175 g) self-raising flour

3 oz (75 g) ground almonds

4 oz (125 g) apricots, chopped

Topping

2 oz (50 g) butter

2 oz (50 g) demerara sugar

1 level teaspoon (8 ml) golden syrup

2 oz (50 g) flaked almonds

Preheat oven: 350°F, 180°C; gas mark 4.

Cream cake butter and sugar together until light, pale and fluffy. Gradually beat in the eggs, adding a tablespoon (15 ml) of flour with each egg. Finally fold in the remaining flour, ground almonds and apricots. Spoon into an 8 in (20 cm) spring clip tin which has been base lined and greased, and level the top. Bake for 45–50 minutes.

While the cake is baking, prepare the topping. Melt the butter, demerara sugar and syrup in a small pan. Heat very gently until the sugar dissolves. Stir in the almonds, spoon over the hot cake and return to the oven for 10–15 minutes to brown.

Apricots are credited with prolonging life and fertility, particularly in the Kashgar region of Pakistan where the fruit is grown in quantity and eaten as a staple part of the diet.

Eat the cake hot as a pudding with yoghurt, or cold for tea. Either way it's delicious.

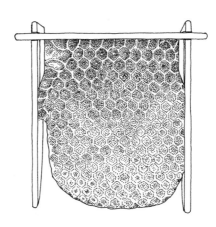

SUSSEX APPLE CAKE

8 oz (225 g) vegetarian margarine
8 oz (225 g) dark brown soft sugar
3 eggs
5 oz (150 g) walnuts
5 oz (150 g) sultanas (or raisins)

8 oz (225 g) self-raising wholemeal
   flour
$\frac{1}{2}$ teaspoon (2.5 ml) ground cloves
14 oz (400 g) cooking apples, peeled and
   chopped

Preheat oven: 350°F, 180°C; gas mark 4.

Grease and base line an 8–9 in (20–23 cm) loose-bottomed tin. Cream together the margarine and 6 oz (175 g) of the sugar. Whip the eggs lightly and beat into the margarine and sugar. Combine 4 oz (125 g) of the crushed walnuts, the sultanas, flour, chopped apples (sliced in a processor or grated) and add cloves.

Put half the cake mixture into the bottom of the tin, then a layer of the fruit and nut mixture and top with the rest of the cake mixture. Sprinkle the remaining 2 oz (50 g) of sugar and 1 oz (25 g) walnuts on top. Bake in oven for $1\frac{1}{2}$ hours.

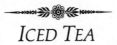

ICED TEA

Ice cubes
Mint

Lemon (or strawberries)

Make a pot of strong tea according to the number of glasses. Fill each glass with ice cubes, add two sprigs of mint and a slice of lemon to each glass – for special occasions sliced fresh strawberries look spectacular. Pour over the tea and serve.

Very refreshing on a hot day.

RUFFORD OLD HALL

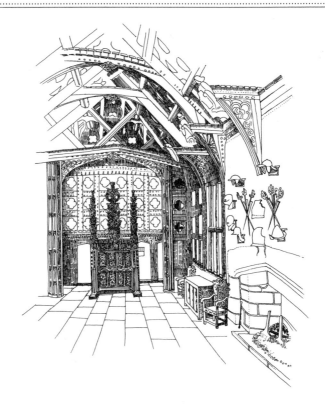

THE only part of the fifteenth-century manor house at Rufford to survive in original form faces visitors coming up the drive: the Great Hall remains the main glory of the house, built on the strength of a series of marriages between the Heskeths and local heiresses. The debt is recorded in the roof bosses of the Great Hall which display the arms of the Lancashire families with which the Heskeths were intermarried, and its elaborate hammer-beam roof supports the stone slates with which the whole house is covered. Below is what is described as a moveable screen, though its size and three finials that almost double its height make it appear anything but portable. It is one of only three remaining in England. The site of the high table, from the time when all members of a household irrespective of rank dined together, is indicated by a canopy of honour and by a great bay window that looks north.

Connecting the Great Hall with a brick Carolean wing is a castellated tower built in 1821 that looms over the earlier parts. The wings incorporates the medieval east wing and its rooms include a large drawing-room with a spy-hole into the Great Hall.

Spread round the house you will find the Philip Ashcroft Collection, everyday items from the nineteenth century. Mr Ashcroft was a member of an old village family still living in Rufford and the first curator of Rufford Old Hall. His collection gives a fascinating insight into the lives of ordinary Lancashire families in the last century. There are carefully worked samplers in the schoolroom, cow creamers, mugs and plates in the tea-room, and in the stables are the larger items – amongst them an enormous cheese press, an early water softener, a frightening mantrap, a towering penny-farthing and a genuine 'boneshaker' bicycle. Exercise was tough stuff. There are pigs in the pig styes, rare bats and bees in the roof and the possibility of a glimpse of the even rarer red squirrel in the beautifully laid-out gardens.

Home-made lunches and teas are served in two delightful small tea-rooms with stone flags, oak furniture and blue-and-white china and linen. Polished pewter and interesting storage jars line the walls, and on chilly days a cheerful fire crackles in the black leaded range. Rufford lies on the flat fertile Lancashire plain, a great area for farming and market gardening. Maureen Dodsworth's recipes reflect the ingredients grown locally, principally vegetables and particularly potatoes, which are famously good in this district. Good 'ribsticking' food to sustain outdoor folk.

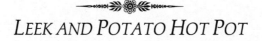

LEEK AND POTATO HOT POT

MAKES FOUR INDIVIDUAL EARTHENWARE DISHES

1 tablespoon (15 ml) sunflower oil	1 teaspoon (5 ml) mustard
1 lb (450 g) leeks	½ pt (250 ml) milk
1lb (450 g) new potatoes, cooked	6 oz (175 g) Cheddar cheese, grated
1½ oz (40 g) butter	parsley, chopped into 1 in (2.5 cm)
1 oz (25 g) plain flour	pieces

Preheat oven: 325°F, 160°C; gas mark 3.

Trim, slice and wash leeks in a colander. Sauté gently in sunflower oil until soft but not mushy. Make a cheese sauce: melt the butter, and stir in and cook the flour for a couple of minutes. Gradually add the milk, stirring all the time, until the mixture comes to the boil and a thick sauce is made. Add the mustard and cheese and heat gently until melted into the sauce.

Arrange half the potatoes in the bottom of each dish, then the leeks, then cover with the cheese sauce. Arrange the balance of the potatoes on top, brush with a little extra oil and bake uncovered in the oven for 20 minutes. Serve with a scattering of chopped parsley.

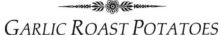

CABBAGE AND POTATO HOT POT

1 lb (450 g) *Savoy cabbage*
1 lb (450 g) *potatoes*
2 *large onions*
4 oz (125 g) *butter or margarine*

1 teaspoon (5 ml) *mixed herbs*
1 teaspoon (5 ml) *ground nutmeg*
salt and pepper

Preheat oven: 425°F, 220°C; gas mark 7.

Slice cabbage and bring to the boil in boiling salted water. Drain in a colander. Peel potatoes and cut into 1/4 in (6 mm) slices. Cook for 5 minutes in boiling water and drain. Slice onions and fry gently in half the butter or margarine until soft but not coloured. Arrange the vegetables in layers in an earthenware dish, seasoning each one. Finish with a layer of potatoes. Dot with the remaining butter and bake in the oven for 30 minutes.

GARLIC ROAST POTATOES

1 *large potato per person*
4 oz (125 g) *butter*
2 *cloves of garlic*

1 tablespoon (15 ml) *of fresh parsley,*
    chopped
1 tablespoon (15 ml) *mixed dried herbs*

Preheat oven: 325°F, 160°C; gas mark 3.

To make the garlic butter, blend the butter, garlic, fresh parsley and mixed dried herbs. This is easily done in a food processor, but you can manage perfectly well with a fork if the butter is soft.

Peel the potatoes, slice in $\frac{1}{4}$ in (6 mm) slices almost through to the base. Melt the garlic butter. Stand each potato on an individual piece of foil large enough to wrap it in. Pour a little butter over each potato, using 1 oz (25 g) garlic butter per person, wrap it in foil and bake for 1 hour.

As well as the wonderful aroma when you unwrap them, you should be able to fan them out, which looks very attractive.

VEGETABLE COBBLER

3 medium carrots, peeled and sliced
½ small cauliflower, separated into
   florets
3 oz (75 g) margarine
8 small leeks, thickly sliced
2 small heads of fennel, sliced

1 oz (25 g) wholewheat flour
¾ pint (400 ml) vegetable stock
salt and pepper
2 tablespoons (30 ml) fresh parsley,
   chopped

Topping

8 oz (225 g) self-raising flour
1 teaspoon (5 ml) mixed herbs
1 teaspoon (5 ml) mustard powder
salt and pepper

2 oz (50 g) vegetarian lard
1 egg
milk to mix
3 oz (75 g) cheese, grated

Preheat oven: 350°F, 180°C; gas mark 4.

Cook carrots and cauliflower for 5 minutes in boiling, salted water and then drain. Place in an ovenproof dish. Melt half the margarine and fry the leeks and fennel over a moderate heat for 3–4 minutes. Add to casserole. Melt the rest of the margarine in a small saucepan, add the wholewheat flour and cook gently for a few minutes. Gradually add the vegetable stock and season if necessary. Simmer for a minute or two, add the parsley and pour over the vegetables. Cover the casserole and bake for 30 minutes.

To make the topping, sieve the flour with the mixed herbs, mustard powder and salt and pepper. Rub in the lard until the mixture resembles coarse breadcrumbs. Mix the egg with a little milk and combine to make a springy dough. Roll out to about ¾ in (2 cm) thick and cut into round scones with a biscuit cutter. Arrange scones on top of the vegetables round the edge of the casserole, sprinkle with the grated cheese. Increase the oven heat to 450°F, 230°C; gas mark 8 and bake the casserole for a further 15 minutes. Serve at once.

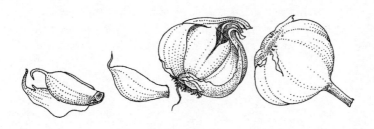

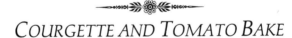

CELERY AND CASHEW NUT RISOTTO

2 tablespoons (30 ml) olive oil or
   sunflower oil
1 onion, finely sliced
4 large sticks of celery, chopped
1 red pepper, diced
8 oz (225 g) brown rice
1 pint (500 ml) vegetable stock
1 dessertspoon (10 ml) oregano

1 tablespoon (15 ml) tomato purée
6 oz (175 g) cashew nuts
1 bunch of spring onions, chopped
1 tablespoon (15 ml) of fresh parsley,
   chopped
2 tablespoons (30 ml) of Parmesan
   cheese, grated

Sauté the chopped onion and celery in the oil in a large frying pan or wok until soft but not brown. Add the red pepper and the rice and stir well so that the rice is well coated with oil. Heat the stock in a small pan, pour one half over the rice mixture and add the oregano and tomato purée. Cover the pan with a lid or foil and simmer until the stock is almost absorbed. Then add the next half together with the cashew nuts and spring onions. Re-cover pan and simmer until the rice is tender. (You may need to top up with a little more stock.) It is important to stir the risotto frequently to ensure that is cooked throughout. Serve with parsley and cheese scattered over the top.

   Olive oil and fresh Parmesan make this a luxurious dish.

COURGETTE AND TOMATO BAKE

2 lb (900 g) courgettes
14 oz (400 g) tin chopped tomatoes
1 teaspoon (5 ml) mixed herbs

2 eggs
$\frac{1}{2}$ pt (250 ml) milk
salt and pepper to taste

Preheat oven: 350°F, 190°C; gas mark 4.

Wash, trim and slice the courgettes. Cook for 5 minutes until not quite tender in boiling water. Drain and layer in the bottom of an ovenproof dish, cover with the chopped tomatoes and herbs and season with pepper and salt. Lightly beat the eggs with the milk, pour over the tomatoes and set the dish uncovered in a roasting tin with water to come half way up the dish. Bake in the oven for about 30 to 40 minutes, until custard is firm.

BRAISED RED CABBAGE

1½ to 2 lb (675–900 g) red cabbage	1 tablespoon (15 ml) vinegar
2 oz (50 g) butter	½ level teaspoon (2 ml) powdered cloves
1 medium-sized onion, sliced	½ teaspoon (2.5 ml) grated nutmeg
1 large cooking apple	freshly ground black pepper, to taste
¼ pt (150 ml) cheap red wine, or stock	1 level tablespoon (13 ml) soft brown
1 dessertspoon (10 ml) salt	sugar

Remove the cabbage's outer leaves, white root and larger pieces of white pith, cut into quarters and shred finely. Place in a large bowl and cover with water. Drain after a minute.

Soften the onions in the melted butter in a large heavy pan, but do not brown. Peel, core and slice thickly the apple, and add to the pan with the wine or stock, salt, vinegar, cloves, nutmeg, plenty of black pepper and finally the cabbage. Combine and cover the pan tightly. Cook gently, stirring occasionally, for about 1 hour, until soft but not mushy. Stir in the sugar and serve.

This loses none of its flavour if reheated the following day.

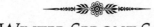

WINTER SPROUT SALAD

1 lb (450 g) sprouts, shredded	½ small head of celery, chopped
½ lb (225 g) carrots, grated	3 oz (75 g) walnuts, broken

Dressing

1 small pot of yoghurt	1 teaspoon (5 ml) seedy mustard
¼ pint (150 ml) mayonnaise	salt and pepper to taste

Combine separately the ingredients of the salad and the dressing. Pour the dressing over the salad. Colourful and crunchy.

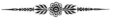

WHOLEMEAL AND YOGHURT SCONES

1 lb (450 g) wholemeal flour
1 teaspoon (5 ml) baking powder
2 oz (50 g) sugar
4 oz (125 g) sultanas

3 oz (75 g) margarine
8 oz (225 ml) natural yoghurt (small
pot)

Preheat oven: 425°F, 220°C; gas mark 7.

Sieve the flour and combine with the baking powder, sugar and sultanas.
Rub in the fat, bind with the yoghurt and cut into rounds. Brush top with
yoghurt and bake in the oven.

Health and Diet

The construction of railways throughout Britain did more to unify
diet and the prices of food than any other development before the
twentieth century. Until towns were linked with the rural hinterland,
a poor harvest in one area could mean hunger and high prices even if
other parts of the country had enjoyed good yields. Equally the
labouring classes in some regions subsisted on food that is now known
to be lacking in nutritional value or of limited help in preventing
degenerative diseases. For example, the staple diet of the poor in the
Midlands and the South was bread, cheese and potatoes washed down
with tea, whereas the barley- or oat-based diet of those in Wales and
the North was much healthier.

The penchant amongst the wealthy for rich food, meat and alcohol
and too few fresh vegetables made gout, heart attacks and cirrhosis of
the liver common ailments. Moreover, the risk of illness from food
was compounded by methods of cooking and food preservation: brass
and copper pans might combine with acid foods to produce poisonous
verdigris, and the failure to boil preserved food in earthenware or
glass jars could cause botulism. The difficulty of keeping food often
meant that ingredients which would today be thrown out as bad were
'rescued' by dubious recipes.

STANDEN

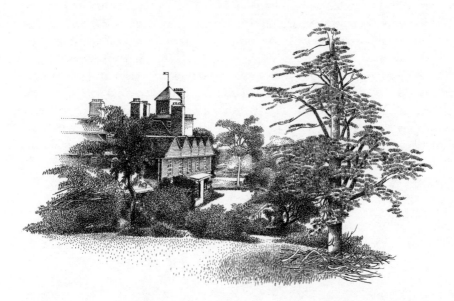

PHILIP WEBB, architect of Standen is quoted as saying: 'I am never satisfied with a design until it begins to look commonplace.' For 'commonplace' read 'a pleasant, commodious, stone Victorian house, beautifully positioned facing south on the North Downs, surrounded by informal gardens and with magnificent views across the River Medway to Ashdown Forest.'

Webb built the house in 1891 for James Beale, a successful solicitor, and his wife Margaret, who wanted a country house for weekends and holidays with their large family. The light airy rooms still convey this relaxed harmonious atmosphere, in total contrast to the cluttered dark rooms normally associated with Victorian interiors.

William Morris, the great nineteenth-century reformer of the decorative arts, was a lifelong friend of Webb, and Morris carpets, wallpapers and fabrics enrich many of the rooms. There is even furniture designed by Morris & Co., such as the seat furniture and the cabinet in the Drawing Room. In other rooms hang original Morris wallpapers and fabrics, now a little faded in contrast with modern copies of original designs that are still on sale today. You will find other great names in the Arts & Crafts movement represented here: glowing, bold pots in red lustre ware by William de Morgan; Della Robbia pottery; pieces of furniture designed by the Misses Garrett; copperware and pottery by John Pearson; brass beds from the fashionable Messrs Heal & Co.; and, of course, various items from the equally fashionable and innovative Messrs Liberty, who are still selling Mr Morris's fabric and wallpaper designs.

Wandering through these rooms and the unpretentious pleasant garden with its lovely views, it is easy to imagine the large Beale family, children, grandchildren and friends enjoying each others' company with conversation and games of billiards inside, promenades and croquet outside. Now Standen invites today's visitors to slow down a little and enjoy the experience of visiting a house and garden which exude the atmosphere of a slower, more leisured age. Standen must have been a pleasure then – it certainly is now.

Turn sharp left by the gate and you will find yourself in an old timber-framed barn. Mrs Simons, the catering manageress, who provided several of the recipes, cooks home-made soups, vegetarian dishes and some lovely cakes. 'I like to keep the individual always in mind. I try to make the visitors feel they are coming to have lunch or tea with me personally.' Philip Webb and the Beales would have approved.

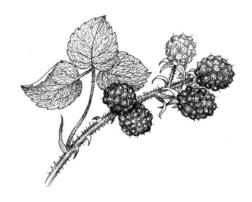

Over-indulgence at Baddesley Clinton
Henry Ferrers of Baddesley Clinton, known as Antiquary Ferrers because of his pursuits in that field, kept a memorandum book most of his life. His diary for 2 November 1622 records: 'had to diner a necke of motton and potage, a piece of powdered biefe and cabage, a leg of goose broyled, a rabbet, a piece of apple tart, cheese, apples and peares ... [Later] I was very sick in the nyghte, and had the sciatica, the collik, and a surfet of the pork in my stomack ...'

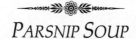

LETTUCE SOUP

1 tablespoon (15 ml) oil

1 oz (25 g) butter

12 oz (350 g) lettuce leaves

1 large leek, sliced

2 medium potatoes, peeled and chopped

1 pt (500 ml) vegetable stock

salt and freshly ground black pepper

parsley, chopped to decorate

Heat the oil and butter in a large saucepan. Tear the lettuce leaves into pieces and sauté in the pan with the sliced leek and chopped potatoes. Pour in the stock, bring to the boil and simmer until the vegetables are tender. Cool slightly before placing in a food processor and processing until smooth. Return to the saucepan and season to taste with salt and pepper. Reheat before serving, ladle into individual bowls and sprinkle over the fresh, chopped parsley.

If you have a row of 'bolting' lettuces (lettuces that are going to seed), this is an excellent recipe to make use of them.

PARSNIP SOUP

1 tablespoon (15 ml) oil

1 oz (25 g) butter

1 medium leek, peeled and sliced

1½ lb (675 g) parsnips, peeled and sliced

1 tablespoon (15 ml) curry powder

2 pt (1.25 l) vegetable stock

salt and freshly ground black pepper

paprika to garnish

Heat the oil and butter in a large saucepan. Sauté the prepared leek and parsnips gently for a few minutes. Stir in the curry powder and continue to cook for a further 2–3 minutes to bring out the flavour. Pour in the stock, bring to the boil and simmer until the vegetables are cooked – approximately 20 minutes. Cool slightly before placing in a food processor and processing until smooth. Return to the saucepan and season to taste with salt and pepper. Reheat before serving, ladle into individual bowls and sprinkle on some paprika.

The touch of curry perfectly complements the nutty flavour of parsnip.

LEEK SOUFFLÉ

3 large eggs, separated
1 lb (450 g) leeks, washed and cut into rings

1 oz (25 g) butter
ground black pepper

Sauce

1 oz (25 g) butter
1 oz (25 g) flour
$\frac{1}{2}$ pt (250 ml) milk

$\frac{1}{4}$ teaspoon (1.25 ml) grated nutmeg
salt and pepper
3 oz (75 g) grated Gruyère cheese

Preheat oven: 375°F, 190°C; gas mark 5.

Grease a 2 pint (1.25 l) soufflé dish.

Separate the eggs. Simmer the leeks in a little boiling water for a few minutes. Drain, add the butter and season.

For the sauce, melt the butter in a saucepan and stir in the flour. Gradually add the milk and bring to the boil, stirring continuously until the sauce thickens. Season with the grated nutmeg and salt and pepper, then stir in the Gruyère cheese.

Stir in the leeks and egg yolks. Whisk the egg whites until stiff and, with a large metal spoon, gently fold them into the soufflé mixture. Pour into the greased soufflé dish and bake for 40–50 minutes until well risen and golden. Serve immediately.

As a main course this serves 3–4, it could also be served as a starter by dividing the mixture between six little ramekins, well-buttered, and baking for 15–20 minutes.

RAISIN AND BRAN LOAF

2 teacups All Bran (cereal)
2 teacups dark brown sugar
2 teacups raisins

2 teacups milk
2 teacups self-raising wholemeal flour

Place the All Bran cereal, sugar, raisins and milk into a pan. Stir, cover and leave overnight.

Preheat oven: 350°F, 180°C; gas mark 4.

Grease and bottom line a 2 lb (900 g) loaf tin.

Add the flour to the mixture; if too stiff, pour in a little more milk or milk and water, to make a soft consistency. Place in the prepared loaf tin and bake in the oven for 45–60 minutes, until a skewer comes out clean. Allow to cool for a few minutes before turning out and removing the lining paper.

Slice and serve spread with butter. A simple but good addition to a high-fibre diet.

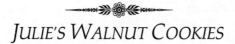

STANDEN GOLDEN CAKE

8 oz (225 g) butter or margarine
8 oz (225 g) caster sugar
3 eggs
8 oz (225 g) carrots, grated

8 oz (225 g) wholemeal self-raising
  flour
4 oz (125 g) sultanas
3 fl oz (75 ml) milk

Preheat oven: 350°F, 180°C; gas mark 4.

Grease and double base line an 8 in (20 cm) cake tin.

Cream together the butter and caster sugar until light and fluffy. Gradually beat in the eggs to the creamed mixture. Stir in the carrots, flour, sultanas and milk, making sure you mix the ingredients well together. Spoon into the prepared tin and bake for 60–70 minutes. Cool in the tin before turning out.

Mrs Simon's Golden Cake is justly famous amongst her customers.

JULIE'S WALNUT COOKIES

8 oz (225 g) butter or margarine
8 oz (225 g) soft brown sugar
$2\frac{1}{2}$ oz (63 g) porridge oats
5 oz (150 g) self-raising flour

2 eggs
4 oz (125 g) chopped walnuts
4 oz (125 g) chopped glacé cherries
$\frac{1}{4}$ teaspoon (1.25 ml) cinnamon

Preheat oven: 350°F, 180°C; gas mark 4.

Grease and line the base of a large Swiss roll tin or smooth-bottomed roasting tin.

Melt the butter in a large saucepan, add the sugar and cook gently until syrupy. Take off the heat and mix in all the other ingredients. Spread evenly over the base of the tin and bake for about 30 minutes.

Take out of the oven and cut into fingers. Leave to cool in the tin.

QUARRY BANK MILL,
STYAL

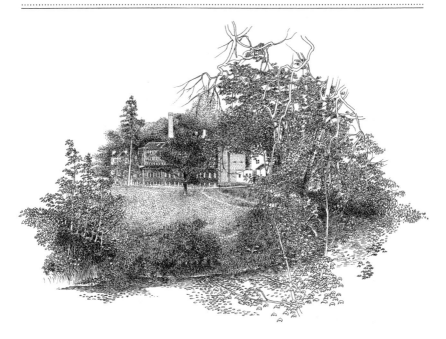

THE Industrial Revolution altered the face of Britain and the lives of millions of people. The huge changes caused by the rise of the great industries of the late eighteenth century – steel, coal and of course, cotton – are still affecting us today. Quarry Bank Cotton Mill at Styal, Cheshire, founded in 1784, was a pioneer factory site of that revolution. Now it is a working museum run by the Quarry Bank Mill Trust.

We are apt to associate industry with grime and ugliness, but at Quarry Bank you will find the human face of the textile trade, set in handsome buildings in a naturally beautiful valley. A mill required power – before the ages of steam and electricity, water provided that power – so at Styal water power was harnessed with pool, weir and headrace from the River Bollin.

Styal is no dusty fusty museum. The experts and enthusiasts you will meet there will bring alive the history of textiles from the early days of spinning and weaving on a hand loom and into the great mechanical weaving sheds. In them 100 per cent cotton calico is still woven today. The cloth is printed with designs exclusive to Styal. Full ranges of clothing, textile products and cloth by the yard are available in the mill shop.

The Greg family who founded Styal built up the business, presided during the great years and later struggled against the changes in demand

and world markets. For two centuries, their lives were inextricably linked with Styal. Samuel Greg and his sons relied largely on poorhouse labour and founded Styal village to house the workforce. By 1790 an Apprentice House was built. Today, like the local schoolchildren, you can experience the hard lives of these 'parish' children. In the whitewashed house are the truckle beds, the desks, slates and pencils, the fustian uniforms, the porridge boiler, even the leeches and potions that the Superintendent used to dose the ailing boys and girls. Long hours, wages of a few shillings a week, crippling fines for misdemeanours, non-existent free time – it all seems draconian now but the Gregs considered themselves good employers by the standards of their time and were proud of their paternalistic labour relations.

Styal calico dresses the windows and dictates the cheerful navy, red and cream colours of the large airy restaurant in the old Weaving Room. No gluey, burnt apprentice porridge here; eat local specialities such as Pan Haggerty and Manchester Tart and enjoy the views towards the weir. The Quarry Bank Mill community is a living example of our industrial heritage.

Apprentice House Recipes

These are not the huge quantities needed to feed 95–100 apprentices of the 1830s.

OATMEAL PORRIDGE

5 pt (2.5 l) of skim	6 tablespoons (90 ml) of oatmeal
2 onions	1 pt (500 ml) of milk or water

Add the onions to the skim and set this to boil. Meanwhile, mix the oatmeal and milk or water until it is very smooth. Pour into the boiling milk and onions. Stir the porridge for 10 minutes, season with salt to taste.

The verdict on this recipe is that it must have tasted awful!

FOR A COUGH SETTLED ON THE STOMACH

$\frac{1}{2}$ lb (225 g) figs, sliced	a stick of liquorice
raisins	few aniseeds and hyssop

Put them all in a quart (1 litre) of spring water. Boil it until it comes to a pint (500 ml), strain and sweeten with sugar. Take $\frac{2}{3}$ spoonful morning and evening or when the cough troubles.

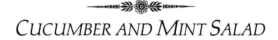

VEGETARIAN MINESTRONE SOUP

2 tablespoons (30 ml) sunflower oil
1 large onion, finely chopped
1 clove of garlic, crushed
3 celery stalks, chopped
2 medium carrots, finely chopped
2 courgettes, finely chopped
14 oz (400 g) tin tomatoes
4 oz (125 g) dried small pasta shells
salt and freshly ground black pepper

1 teaspoon (5 ml) oregano
1 teaspoon (5 ml) sugar
1 tablespoon (15 ml) tomato purée
$2\frac{1}{2}$ pt (1.5 l) vegetable stock
1 medium tin white haricot beans,
    rinsed and drained
4 oz (125 g) Parmesan cheese, grated,
    to garnish

Heat the oil in a heavy-based saucepan and sauté the onion and garlic gently until soft. Stir in the remaining vegetables (except the beans) and pasta. Add salt and pepper to taste, stir in the herbs, sugar, tomato purée and stock. Bring to the boil, stirring frequently. Lower the heat, cover and simmer gently for 20 minutes stirring occasionally. Add the beans and pasta shells and simmer for a further 10 minutes or until the vegetables are tender. Adjust the seasonings and serve piping hot with the Parmesan handed round separately.

A main course soup to satisfy hearty appetites.

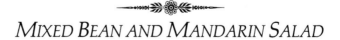

CUCUMBER AND MINT SALAD

1 large cucumber, cubed
mint, chopped, to taste

5 oz (150 g) carton thick natural
    yoghurt

Wash and cut the cucumber into 1 in (2.5 cm) cubes and place in a decorative glass bowl. If using fresh mint, bruise the leaves and chop finely. Add to the yoghurt to taste. If using concentrated mint from a jar, about 1 heaped teaspoon (6 ml) should be sufficient. Stir the mint into the yoghurt, then pour over the cucumber and toss to combine. Cover and leave in the fridge for about 45 minutes for the flavours to marinate before serving.

MIXED BEAN AND MANDARIN SALAD

1 medium tin red kidney beans
1 small tin mandarins in own juice

4 oz (125 g) cooked broad beans
salt and freshly ground black pepper

Thoroughly rinse the kidney beans and drain. Drain the juice from the mandarins and reserve. Combine the kidney beans, broad beans and mandarins in a salad bowl, season with a little salt and black pepper and toss lightly with a little of the mandarin juice.

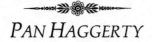

PAN HAGGERTY

1 lb (450 g) potatoes
8 oz (225 g) onions
1 tablespoon (15 ml) white Flora (or butter)

4 oz (125 g) Lancashire cheese, grated
salt and pepper

Slice the potatoes and onions very thinly. Heat the Flora in a large non-stick frying pan and put in the potatoes and onions with the grated cheese in layers, seasoning each layer lightly with salt and pepper. Fry it all gently until cooked. Place in an ovenproof casserole dish and brown under a grill.

This makes a delicious supper dish served with a crisp, green salad.

LEEK AND PARSNIP BAKE

1 tablespoon (15 ml) vegetable oil
4 washed leeks, chopped into chunks
1 lb (450 g) parsnips, sliced
3 oz (75 g) butter
2 oz (50 g) plain flour

1 teaspoon (5 ml) mustard
$\frac{3}{4}$ pt (400 ml) milk
8 oz (225 g) cheese, grated
2 or 3 sticks of celery
flaked almonds

Preheat oven: 375°F, 190°C; gas mark 5.

Heat the oil gently in a large frying pan and sauté the leeks and parsnips until cooked but still slightly crunchy. Divide the vegetables evenly among 4 individual gratin dishes. Make a cheese sauce: melt the butter in a saucepan, stir in the flour with a teaspoon of mustard and cook for a minute or two before pouring in the milk. Stirring all the time, bring to the boil, then add 6 oz (175 g) of the grated cheese.

Pour the cheese sauce over the vegetables and mix lightly together to combine the ingredients. Slice the sticks of celery *very thinly*. Sprinkle the remaining grated cheese over each dish followed by the sliced celery and top with flaked almonds. Bake in the oven for 15 minutes until lightly golden on top.

LANCASHIRE CHEESE AND ONION TART

8 oz (225 g) shortcrust pastry
2 medium onions
2 oz (50 g) butter
12 oz (350 g) Lancashire cheese, grated

1 egg, beaten
2 fl oz (60 ml) milk
salt and pepper
2 large tomatoes

Line an 8–9 in (20–23 cm) flan dish with shortcrust pastry and chill in the fridge while preparing the other ingredients. Chop the onions and sauté in the butter until transparent. Place them evenly over the pastry and fill the flan with the grated cheese. Mix together the beaten egg and milk and season with salt and pepper. Pour this into the pastry case. Slice 2 tomatoes and arrange in a circle around the edge of the pie. Stand the tin on a baking tray and bake for 30 minutes or until the pastry is cooked and the filling is a golden brown and firm to touch (not sloppy in the middle). Serve hot with a salad of your choice.

Lancashire cheese has long been considered one of the best English cheeses for cooking.

MANCHESTER HOT CAKES

1 oz (25 g) butter
1 oz (25 g) vegetarian lard
8 oz (225 g) self-raising flour

1 tablespoon (15 ml) caster sugar
1 egg
milk to mix

Preheat oven: 425°F, 220°C; gas mark 7.

Lightly grease a baking sheet. Rub the fats into the flour using your fingertips. Next stir in the sugar. Beat the egg and, using a knife, mix it into the flour with a little milk to make a soft dough. Knead gently with your hands, then turn out on to a floured pastry board. Roll out to a thickness of not less than $\frac{3}{4}$ in (2 cm) and cut into rounds using a $1\frac{1}{2}$–2 in (4–5 cm) pastry cutter. Place on the greased baking sheet and bake near the top of a hot oven for 12–15 minutes until nicely brown. Butter and serve hot.

Must be eaten while hot and fresh as they can go stale very quickly.

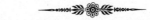

MANCHESTER TART

6 oz (175 g) shortcrust pastry (use the
Mulberry and Apple Pie recipe from
Moseley, p. 107, using half the
ingredients)
2 tablespoons (30 ml) strawberry jam

1 pt (500 ml) custard (commercial
custard tastes best!)
1 heaped tablespoon (17 ml) dessicated
coconut

Preheat oven: 400°F, 200°C; gas mark 6.

Line a 7 in (18 cm) flan tin with the shortcrust pastry, prick well and bake
blind for 20 minutes until the pastry has set, removing the beans 6–7
minutes before the end of the cooking time. The pastry should be an even,
light golden brown colour.

Allow to cool before spreading the strawberry jam over the base of the
pastry, then pour over the prepared custard (the custard should be of a nice,
smooth consistency as one would use for trifle). Sprinkle a little dessicated
coconut over the custard and leave to cool.

Serve cold with whipped cream.

OLD HANNAH'S CHESHIRE POTATO CAKES

8 oz (225 g) self-raising flour
$\frac{1}{2}$ teaspoon (2.5 ml) salt
2 oz (50 g) butter or margarine
8 oz (225 g) left-over mashed potatoes
or fresh

1 egg, beaten
a little milk if required

Preheat oven: 375°F, 190°C; gas mark 5.

Grease a baking tray. Place the flour and salt in a bowl with the fat. Rub the
fat in the flour using your fingertips, then fork in the mashed potatoes.

Make a well in the centre of the mixture and drop in the beaten egg. Fork
it into the mixture using a little milk if necessary, to give a soft pliable
dough. Finish by kneading the dough with your hands until smooth. Roll it
out to approximately $\frac{1}{2}$ in (1.25 cm) thick and cut into rounds with a pastry
cutter. Space them out on the prepared baking sheet and bake for 30
minutes.

Take out of the oven and wrap in a clean tea towel to keep them warm
and soft. Split, butter and spread them with jam or syrup and serve while
hot. Leftover cakes can be reheated, but they will have a crispy surface.

BANANA BREAD

4 oz (125 g) butter or soft margarine	1 heaped teaspoon (6 ml) baking
4 oz (125 g) caster sugar	powder
8 oz (225 g) mashed bananas (overripe	$\frac{1}{4}$ teaspoon (1.25 ml) bicarbonate of
bananas are particularly suitable)	soda
1 egg, lightly beaten	$\frac{1}{4}$ teaspoon (1.25 ml) salt
7 oz (200 g) plain flour	$\frac{1}{4}$ teaspoon (1.25 ml) vanilla essence

Preheat oven: 350°F, 180°C; gas mark 4.

Grease and line a 1 lb (450 g) loaf tin.

Cream together the butter and sugar until light and fluffy. Stir in the mashed bananas and the beaten egg; do not worry if the mixture looks curdled at this stage.

Gradually fold in the sieved, dry ingredients and the vanilla essence. Spoon into the prepared loaf tin and bake for 45–50 minutes, until the cake springs back when lightly pressed with a finger.

Cool in the tin for 10 minutes before turning out on to a wire rack to cool completely.

Serve this loaf cake sliced thickly and buttered. It freezes well.

STYAL CARROT CAKE

6 oz (175 g) carrots, grated	2 eggs, lightly beaten
4 oz (125 g) walnuts, chopped	6 oz (175 g) wholemeal flour
6 oz (175 g) soft brown sugar	1 teaspoon (5 ml) cinnamon
6 oz (175 g) corn oil	1 teaspoon (5 ml) bicarbonate of soda

Topping

2 oz (50 g) soft margarine	3 oz (75 g) sifted icing sugar
6 oz (175 g) cream cheese	walnuts to decorate
rind $\frac{1}{2}$ lemon, grated	

Preheat oven: 350°F, 180°C; gas mark 4.

Grease and bottom line an 8 in (20 cm) cake tin. Grate the washed and peeled carrots and finely chop the walnuts. Mix together in a basin with the soft brown sugar. Stir in the corn oil and the two beaten eggs and mix thoroughly together.

Stir together the wholemeal flour, cinnamon and bicarbonate of soda and fold these dry ingredients into the carrot mixture, lightly but thoroughly.

Spoon into the prepared tin and bake for approximately 50 minutes. The cake is cooked when it springs back when lightly pressed with a finger. Leave to cool in the tin for a few minutes, then turn out on to a wire rack.

Make the topping by creaming together the margarine and cream cheese until light and fluffy. Stir the lemon rind into the icing sugar and gradually beat this into the creamed mixture until all the sugar is incorporated.

When the cake is cold spread the topping over the top of the cake and decorate with chopped walnuts. Store in the fridge.

Dr Peter Holland was doctor to the apprentices at Styal from 1795 to 1837, and the Mill still has his notebooks. The apprentices were healthy by the standards of their time. Samuel Greg ensured this by insisting that any children supplied to him by parish authorities should come on a trial period of a month 'to ascertain their probable healthiness'. In practice, the system was more relaxed. Notes for 28 February 1833 state: 'Sarah Powell, Liverpool, aged 9. Healthy now. Had inflamed eyes a year ago but they are well now, and there does not seem any objection to engaging her.'

Many of the health problems were work-related: sore eyes, headaches, cuts, bruises. Accidents were not often recorded.

Dr Holland's 'science' consisted of four humours medicine – bad body fluid caused any number of infections and health problems. Leeches were used to take away bad blood. For instance, Elizabeth Bracegirdle was treated for inflamed eyes in November 1841: 'four leeches round the right eye and in three days a blister behind the right ear, to be repeated in five or six days.'

Here are some interesting facts about leeches generously supplied by the Apprentice House: each leech has 300 teeth and 3 jaws; a leech can take 8fl oz (225 ml) blood (if the doctor snipped the tail, it would take more, but it would also die); they can gorge feed every six months. In 1830, the leeches for Styal probably came from the River Bollin, but leech gatherers also collected them from the Lake District. Doctors could 'drain' leeches by putting them in a bowl of hot water and pressing the blood out of them. Leeches are being used again in hospitals to aid micro-surgery.

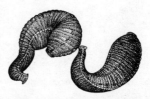

WALLINGTON

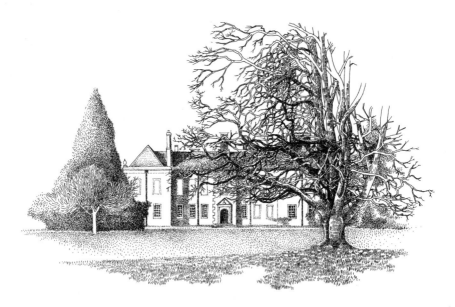

RIVE north east across the bleak, beautiful Northumbrian moors from Newcastle and suddenly, over the brow of a hill, Wallington appears below, a grey Palladian mansion, approached across a handsome bridge and guarded by four huge stone griffins' heads. (They once adorned one of the entrances to the City of London, Bishopsgate.)

Since 1688 Wallington has belonged first to the Blackett and later the Trevelyan families. Both had a tradition of public service. Throughout the centuries, Blacketts and Trevelyans served as Mayors of Newcastle and Members of Parliament. Although permanently short of money, Walter Calverley Blackett, whose portrait by Reynolds hangs in the Saloon, remodelled the house, built the stable block and created a beautiful walled valley garden, reached by a walk through woods that he planted.

All the Trevelyans were cultured and well read: in the well-stocked library you will find books annotated with amusingly barbed hand-written comments. They were also historians; Lord Macaulay, whose desk is in the house, was related by marriage, and dedicated to social reform. This was particularly true of Walter and Pauline Trevelyan, Victorian owners of Wallington. Walter was very interested in natural history, agriculture and the temperance movement: his signature, with Pauline's, appears on a tract against 'ardent spirits' quoted opposite. Pauline was deeply involved with the pre-Raphaelite brotherhood, and was herself a talented painter. With a little help from John Ruskin, she and William Bell Scott created the huge allegorical pictures of Northumbrian history in the central hall. Although committed teetotallers – there are no public houses still on the Wallington estate – Pauline did persuade Walter to relax a little as far as house guests were concerned and table wine of doubtful quality was provided. One house guest, however, was not to be mollified by this gesture: Augustus Hare, who stayed at Wallington in 1861 and 1862. On his first visit he arrived for lunch 'which was as peculiar as everything else (Lady Trevelyan and her artists feeding solely on artichokes and cauliflowers)'. On his second visit he sourly described the house 'like a great desert with one or two oases', though he ended up enjoying himself because of the excellent conversation of his hosts. Life with Walter and Pauline must have been interesting but uncomfortable.

Now things are ordered better. Allow time to see the elegant eighteenth-century interiors, particularly the porcelain, a village of doll's-houses and armies of lead soldiers and the Victorian kitchen. Upstairs is a pretty nursery, bedrooms full of family pictures and furniture and Lady Wilson's Cabinet of Curiosities – a room of glass cases, with the strangest mixture of objects: stuffed birds, eggs and minerals jostle with models, utensils, photographs and ephemera, designed to startle, intrigue and amaze the beholder.

Walk the woods, stroll in the sheltered valley garden and cross the grassy quadrangle to eat hearty Northumbrian food in the beamed Clocktower Restaurant. Northumbrians are proud of their leeks, and the soup and pudding given here would keep out the chill of the coldest winter day. Home-made biscuits are another speciality, easy to make and a treat to eat.

This notice hangs in the room containing the doll's-house at Wallington:

ASSOCIATION FOR THE SUPPRESSION OF INTEMPERANCE

We the subscribers agree, so long as we belong to this Association, to abstain from the use of ardent spirits except for medicinal purposes, and to refrain from providing them for persons in our employ.

Signed by amongst others John Trevelyan
Pauline Trevelyan
Arthur Trevelyan
W. C. Trevelyan, all of Wallington

1831–34

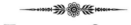

LEEK AND POTATO BROTH

$1\frac{1}{2}$ lb (675 g) potatoes
1 oz (25 g) butter
$\frac{1}{2}$ pint (250 ml) milk

1 lb (450 g) leeks
salt and pepper
pinch of nutmeg

Peel the potatoes and boil until soft. Drain and mash into creamed potato with the butter and milk. Prepare and chop the leeks, just cover with water in a saucepan, season with salt and cook until tender. Combine the creamed potato with the leeks and the cooking water and season to taste with salt and pepper and a pinch of nutmeg. Serve piping hot.

This is a creamy soup and filling enough for a main meal.

TROPICAL SALAD

2 tomatoes
1 red apple
1 green apple
1 small pepper
8 oz (225 g) mixed green and black grapes

1 large orange
3 thick slices cucumber
1 banana
$\frac{1}{4}$ pint (150 ml) white wine vinegar

Chop, slice or dice, according to your personal preference, all the fruit and salad ingredients. Pour over the wine vinegar and chill before serving.

An excellent recipe for slimmers.

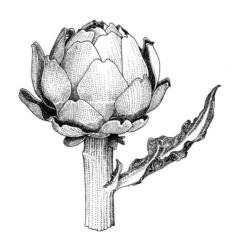

Although Pauline Trevelyan's fare of artichokes and cauliflowers may have been sparse, that of an earlier owner of Wallington certainly was not. Mary Smith, formerly housekeeper to Sir William Blackett of Wallington, went on to write in 1772 *The Complete Housekeeper*, in which she provided suggested bills of fare for the months of the year. For February, which might be considered a lean month of the calendar, her recommendations were:

First Course   Soupe la reine removed with turbot; Fowl broiled with mushroom sauce; Pigeon cutlets; Lobster sauce; Veal pie; Pickles; Fricasee of sheep trotters the Italian way; Anchovy sauce; Mutton collops; Roast Beef.

Second Course   Three partridges roasted; White pot pudding; Preserved oranges in quarters; Pigeons; Preserved pineapple; Prawns; Whipt posset; Preserved ginger; Preserved raspberries; Preserved currant tart; Collared pig; Four sweetbreads roasted.

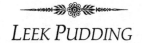

LEEK PUDDING

8 oz (225 g) self-raising flour
$\frac{1}{2}$ teaspoon (2.5 ml) salt
4 oz (125 g) vegetarian suet
about 8 tablespoons (120 ml) water

$1\frac{1}{4}$ lb (550 g) leeks
herbs of your choice (optional)
salt and pepper

Preheat oven: 350°F, 180°C; gas mark 4.

Mix together the flour, salt and suet. Add enough water to produce a light, elastic dough and knead gently until smooth. Roll into a rectangle approximately $\frac{1}{4}$ in (6 mm) thick. Chop the leeks and sprinkle on to the pastry, leaving a margin round the edges. If you wish add some herbs and season with salt and pepper. Roll up like a Swiss roll and seal the ends with your fingers.

Lightly butter a piece of tinfoil and wrap up the roll, not too tightly to allow for expansion. Bake in the oven for approximately $1\frac{1}{2}$ hours or until the pastry is golden and cooked through. This is delicious served with a vegetable stew such as ratatouille (see Montacute p. 98).

SHERRY FRUIT SLICE

1 lb (450 g) shortcrust pastry (made
with $\frac{3}{4}$ vegetarian lard to $\frac{1}{4}$
margarine for extra crispness); a
recipe is given on p. 107
1 cooking apple, grated

8 oz (225 g) mixed dried fruit (sultanas,
raisins, currants)
1 oz (25 g) butter
1 small wine glass medium or sweet
sherry
juice of half a lemon

Preheat oven: 400°F, 200°C; gas mark 6.

Line a 10 in (25 cm) pie plate with half the pastry. Spread the grated apple
over the pastry. Bring the fruit, butter, sherry and lemon juice to the boil,
allow to cool a little and spread the mixture over the apple. Then roll out
the rest of the pastry and cover the pie, sealing the edges with a little milk.
Cut air holes in the top, brush with milk and bake for 30 minutes until the
pastry is cooked and golden brown.

Good, hot, warm or cold.

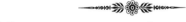

NORTHUMBRIAN APPLE STRUDEL

8 oz (225 g) self-raising flour
$\frac{1}{2}$ teaspoon (2.5 ml) salt
4 oz (125 g) vegetarian suet
about 8 tablespoons (120 ml) water
1 lb (450 g) cooking apples, sliced

3 tablespoons (45 ml) mincemeat
$\frac{1}{4}$ teaspoon (2.5 ml) cinnamon
1 tablespoon (15 ml) soft brown sugar
a little milk

Preheat oven: 350°F, 180°C; gas mark 4.

Mix together the flour, salt and suet. Add enough water to produce a
light, elastic dough and knead gently until smooth. Roll into a rectangle
approximately $\frac{1}{4}$ in (6 mm) thick. Spread the apple slices and the mincemeat
evenly over the pastry, leaving a margin round the edges. Scatter over it
the cinnamon and sugar. Roll up like a Swiss roll and seal the ends with a
little milk.

Lightly butter a piece of tinfoil and wrap up, not too tightly to allow for
expansion. Bake in the oven for approximately $1\frac{1}{2}$ hours or until the pastry
is golden and cooked through.

Serve warm, cut in slices with cream or yoghurt.

CHOCOLATE PEANUT BISCUITS

4 oz (125 g) butter
5 oz (150 g) brown sugar
2 eggs

6 oz (175 g) self-raising flour
1 oz (25 g) cocoa powder
8 oz (225 g) unsalted peanuts, chopped

Preheat oven: 350°F, 180°C; gas mark 4.

Grease two baking sheets. Cream together the butter and sugar until light and fluffy. Gradually beat in the eggs. Gently fold into the mixture the flour, cocoa powder and coarsely chopped peanuts. Place small spoonfuls on to the baking sheets and flatten slightly. Bake in the oven for around 15 minutes, then place on a wire rack to cool.

WHITTINGHAM BUTTONS

6 oz (175 g) butter or margarine
3 oz (75 g) icing sugar

6 oz (175 g) plain flour
2 oz (50 g) custard powder

Preheat oven: 350°F, 180°C; gas mark 4.

Cream the butter and sugar together very thoroughly until light and fluffy. Add the flour and custard powder and mix to form a firm dough. Break off small pieces, the size of a large walnut, and roll into a ball with your hands or place small spoonfuls on to a greased baking sheet and flatten slightly. Bake in a preheated oven for 10–15 minutes or until lightly golden. Cool on a wire rack.

This is a local recipe; Whittingham is only a few miles away.

WIMPOLE HALL

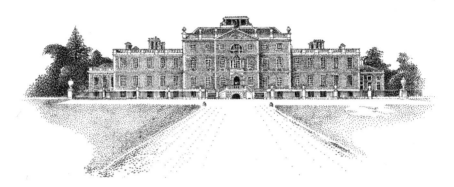

WIMPOLE, the largest house in Cambridgeshire, is set with church, stables and home farm in a great park of mature trees, lakes, avenues and statuary. A romantic Gothick tower ruin, built in 1768 by Capability Brown, enhances the view from the house. Brown was only one of the celebrated architects and landscape gardeners who 'altered and improved' Sir Thomas Chicheley's original designs. James Gibbs, Charles Bridgeman, Henry Flitcroft, Sir John Soane, Humphry Repton and H. E. Kendall all contributed too. Today their achievement is an astonishingly harmonious blend of buildings and landscape.

Cambridgeshire is a countryside of gently rolling fields, tall trees and huge skies. Views are on the grand scale and so is Wimpole. Although the interiors are appropriately imposing, they are not overpowering. The last private owner of the house, Elsie Bambridge, Rudyard Kipling's daughter, died as recently as 1976. During her time at Wimpole, she furnished and decorated the house, filling it with pictures; her love and concern remains a strong influence. Through the tall windows the clear East Anglian light reflects fine carving, plasterwork and gilding, and illuminated, elegant, unfussy rooms. To me, the most beautiful of all is Sir John Soane's Yellow Drawing Room, lit from a painted dome, a wonderfully appropriate setting for the grand occasions of eighteenth-century country life. He also built a plunge bath where jaded gentry dipped for cleanliness rather than health!

James Gibbs' magnificent Baroque chapel inside the house may have been built as a suitable setting for performances by the orchestra kept by the then owner of Wimpole, Lord Harley. In complete contrast is the Wimpole parish church of St Andrew's, small and intimate, and full of marble monuments to the Yorke family* who owned Wimpole for over a hundred years. Beyond the church is H. E. Kendall's Victorian stables where a wagon ride can be taken to Sir John Soane's other contribution to

Wimpole, the Home Farm buildings. Here the Rare Breeds Survival Trust is raising old strains of cattle, sheep, goats and other livestock, providing not only an opportunity to see these animals but also to make a positive contribution to farm-stock breeding in the future.

Feast in style at Wimpole, below the chandeliers and gilded plasterwork of the original Great Dining Room. Splendid views across the park enhance the fresh delicious dishes flavoured with herbs from the garden. Food for fitness is a speciality here; the restaurant is rightly proud of its Heartbeat Award won for low-fat/high-fibre meals. All the recipes from Wimpole are appetising and interesting; I'm sure they will tempt the most reluctant convert to healthy eating.

*The Yorke family at Erddig was related, pp. 76–8.

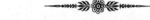

WIMPOLE'S GREEK SALAD

12 oz (350 g) tomatoes, cut into
    quarters
½ cucumber, unpeeled and chopped
½ large mild onion, sliced and chopped
6 oz (175 g) mature Cheddar, cut into
    small cubes

12 black olives
black pepper
5 tablespoons (75 ml) olive oil
½ teaspoon (2.5 ml) dried oregano

Pile the tomatoes, cucumber and onion in a large salad bowl. Scatter over the cubes of cheddar cheese, add the olives, sprinkle with black pepper and dress with olive oil. Scatter oregano over the top.

The oregano is absolutely essential for an authentic Greek flavour.

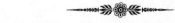

WILD AND BROWN RICE SALAD

1 oz (25 g) butter
8 oz (225 g) brown rice
2 oz (50 g) wild rice
1¼ pints (750 ml) boiling water or stock
1 teaspoon (5 ml) salt

5 tablespoons (75 ml) vinaigrette
    dressing
1 small green pepper
1 small red pepper
1 small tin kidney beans
bunch spring onions, chopped

Heat the butter in a saucepan, then stir in the rice so that it gets nicely coated with the butter. Add the boiling water (or stock) and salt, stir once only, then cover and simmer gently for 40 minutes or until all the liquid has been absorbed. Tip the rice into a salad bowl and fluff it up with a fork. Pour over the dressing while it is still warm. Leave it to get cold, then mix in all the other ingredients, adding more dressing if necessary and salt and pepper.

CURRIED CABBAGE BAKE

1 medium cabbage (Primo or similar)

Sauce

1 small onion

2 tablespoons (30 ml) oil

2 tablespoons (30 ml) curry powder

1 tablespoon (15 ml) flour

1 dessertspoon (10 ml) tomato purée

1 oz (25 g) creamed coconut

2 tablespoons (30 ml) mango chutney

$\frac{3}{4}$ pint (400 ml) vegetable stock (use the water from the cabbage with an added stock cube)

salt and pepper

Topping

2 oz (50 g) hazelnuts, finely chopped

2 oz (50 g) bread-crumbs

$\frac{1}{2}$ teaspoon (2.5 ml) cumin seeds

1 teaspoon (5 ml) sesame seeds

Cut the cabbage into six wedges, place in a large saucepan and cover with water. Bring to the boil and simmer until just tender (about 15 minutes). Drain, reserving the cabbage water, and arrange in an ovenproof dish. Cover and keep warm.

Make the curry sauce as follows: chop the onion and sauté in the oil until soft. Stir in the curry powder and flour and cook for a further minute or two stirring all the time. Add the tomato purée, creamed coconut, mango chutney and vegetable stock and bring to the boil. Simmer gently for 5–10 minutes, season to taste with salt and pepper, then coat the segments of cabbage with the sauce.

Mix together all the topping ingredients and scatter over the top. Place the dish under a hot grill until brown and crispy. Serve immediately.

This is a rich, filling dish and needs only relishes such as cucumber raita or tomato and onion to accompany it.

MUSHROOM STROGANOFF

1 medium onion, finely chopped	$\frac{1}{4}$ teaspoon (2.5 ml) dried or fresh thyme
2 sticks celery, finely sliced	$\frac{1}{2}$ pint (250 ml) vegetable stock
half medium red pepper, chopped	1 level dessertspoon (8 ml) cornflour
half medium green pepper, chopped	salt and pepper
2 oz (50 g) butter	12 oz (350 g) button mushrooms
1 bayleaf	1 small pot yoghurt

Sauté in a large saucepan the onion, celery and peppers in 1 oz (25 g) butter, stirring now and again, for about 5 minutes. Add the herbs, vegetable stock and bring to the boil. Simmer for 10 minutes, until the vegetables are cooked. In a cup mix the cornflour with a little cold water to make a cream and add to the pan to thicken the stock. Season well with salt and freshly ground black pepper.

Wipe the button mushrooms if necessary, toss in the remaining butter until barely cooked and add to the sauce. Just before serving, heat through gently until piping hot, then stir in the yoghurt.

Serve on a bed of brown rice, or, for a special occasion, a mixture of wild rice and brown.

STUFFED MUSHROOMS

8 large flat mushrooms (if very large allow one per person)	4 oz (125 g) bread-crumbs
	4 oz (125 g) cheese, grated
2 tablespoons (30 ml) olive oil	$\frac{1}{4}$ teaspoon (1.25 ml) fresh thyme
1 onion, finely chopped	1 tablespoon (15 ml) parsley, chopped
2 cloves of garlic, crushed	1 egg, beaten
1 oz (25 g) butter	salt and pepper

Preheat oven: 425°F, 220°C; gas mark 7.

Remove and reserve any stems from the mushrooms. Brush the mushrooms with the oil and place them in a single layer in a large baking dish or on a baking tray. Bake them in the hot oven for five minutes.

Sauté the chopped onion and garlic in the butter together with the stems from the mushrooms, finely chopped. Place in a mixing bowl and add the bread-crumbs, 2 oz (50 g) of grated cheese, thyme and parsley. Mix well together and combine with the beaten egg. Season with salt and pepper and fill each mushroom cap with the mixture. Sprinkle on the balance of the cheese and return to the oven for 15 minutes, until the top is golden.

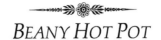

BEANY HOT POT

4 oz (125 g) dried flagelot beans
4 oz (125 g) dried chick peas
2½ pints (1.5 l) vegetable stock
14 oz (400 g) tin red kidney beans

1 dessertspoon (10 ml) tomato purée
1 teaspoon (5 ml) mixed herbs
salt and pepper

Topping
2 oz (50 g) cheese, grated
2 oz (50 g) fresh brown bread-crumbs

salt and pepper

Soak the dried pulses overnight and then drain.

Preheat oven: 375°F, 190°C; gas mark 5.

Cook the drained pulses separately in the stock. Place ¾ of the pulses and all the tinned red kidney beans (drained and rinsed), into a casserole, reserving any cooking liquid. If necessary, make up the cooking liquid to ¾ pint (400 ml) and blend with the balance of the pulses in a food processor. Return to a saucepan and stir in the tomato purée, mixed herbs and seasoning. Heat until boiling, then pour into the casserole with the beans.

Mix the cheese and bread-crumb topping and spread in a thick layer on top. Cook uncovered for 20 minutes until the top is crisp and golden.

Sir John Soane designed the plunge bath at Wimpole for the 3rd Earl of Hardwicke in 1792. In the eighteenth century, dips in cold water, preferably mineral springs, were regarded as efficacious against headaches, impotence and sundry other maladies. Bath, of course, was a great social centre at the time, but gentlemen often wished to continue the treatments on their return to their country homes. Usually bath-houses were placed in parks, away from the house (see Kedleston Hall, p. 85) but Wimpole is a rare and handsome instance of an indoor bath.

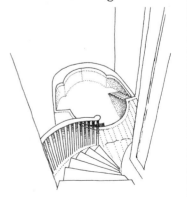

NATIONAL TRUST
RESTAURANTS

AVON

Dyrham Park
Unlicensed tea-room
The Orangery, Dyrham Park,
Chippenham
Tel: (027582) 2501

BERKSHIRE

Basildon Park
Unlicensed tea-room
Lower Basildon, Reading
Tel: (07357) 3040

Cliveden
Unlicensed restaurant
Taplow, Maidenhead
Tel: (06286) 61406

BUCKINGHAMSHIRE

Claydon House
Unlicensed tea-room
Middle Claydon, Nr Buckingham
Tel: (029673) 349 or 693

Hughenden Manor
Unlicensed tea-room
High Wycombe
Tel: (0494) 32580

CAMBRIDGESHIRE

Anglesey Abbey
Licensed restaurant
Lode, Cambridge
Tel: (0223) 811200

Peckover House
Unlicensed tea-room
North Brink, Wisbech
Tel: (0945) 583463

Wimpole Hall
Licensed restaurant

Wimpole Home Farm House
Unlicensed refreshments
Arrington, Nr Royston,
Hertfordshire
Tel: (0223) 207257

CHESHIRE

Dunham Massey
Licensed restaurant
Altrincham
Tel: (061941) 1025

Little Moreton Hall
Unlicensed tea-room
Congleton
Tel: (0260) 272018

CLEVELAND

Ormesby Hall
Light refreshments
Ormesby, Middlesbrough
Tel: (0642) 324188

CORNWALL

Bedruthan Steps
Unlicensed café
St Eval, Wadebridge
Tel: (0637) 860563

Cotehele
Licensed restaurant
St Dominick, Saltash
Tel: (0579) 50652

Unlicensed restaurant
The Edgcumbe Arms
The Quay, Cotehele,
St Dominick
Tel: (0579) 50024

Lanhydrock
Licensed restaurant
Lanhydrock Park, Bodmin
Tel: (0208) 4331

St Michael's Mount
Licensed restaurant
The Sail Loft Restaurant
St Michael's Mount, Marazion,
Penzance
Tel: (0736) 710748

Trelissick Garden
Licensed restaurant
Feock, Truro
Tel: (0872) 863486

Trerice
Licensed restaurant
St Newlyn East, Newquay
Tel: (0637) 875404

CUMBRIA

Fell Foot
Unlicensed café
Fell Foot Park, Newby Bridge,
Ulverston
Tel: (053 95) 31273

Sizergh Castle
Unlicensed tea-room
Nr Kendal
Tel: (05395) 60070

Wordsworth House
Licensed restaurant
Main Street, Cockermouth
Tel: (0900) 824805

DERBYSHIRE

Hardwick Hall
Licensed restaurant
Doe Lea, Chesterfield
Tel: (0246) 850430

Kedleston Hall
Licensed restaurant
Kedleston, Derby
Tel: (0332) 842191

Longshaw Lodge
Unlicensed café
Longshaw, Sheffield
Tel: (0433) 31708

Sudbury Hall
Unlicensed restaurant
Sudbury Coach House, Sudbury
Tel: (028378) 597

DEVON

Arlington Court
Licensed restaurant
Arlington, Nr Barnstaple
Tel: (027 182) 348

Castle Drogo
Licensed restaurant
Drewsteignton, Exeter
Tel: (06473) 3306

Killerton
Licensed restaurant
Broadclyst, Exeter
Tel: (0392) 881345

Knightshayes Court
Licensed restaurant
Bolham, Tiverton
Tel: (0884) 254665

Saltram
Licensed restaurant
Plympton, Plymouth
Tel: (0752) 336546

Watersmeet House
Unlicensed tea-room
Lynmouth
Tel: (0598) 3348

DORSET

Brownsea Island
Licensed café
Café Villano, Brownsea Island,
Poole Harbour
Tel: (0202) 700244

Corfe Castle
Licensed tea-room
Castle Tea-room, Corfe Castle, Nr
Wareham
Tel: (0929) 480921

Kingston Lacy
Unlicensed restaurant
Wimborne Minster
Tel: (0202) 883402

EAST SUSSEX

Bateman's
Licensed tea-room
Burwash, Etchingham
Tel: (0435) 882302

Bodiam Castle
Licensed café
Bodiam, Nr Robertsbridge
Tel: (058083) 436

GLOUCESTERSHIRE

Hidcote Manor Garden
Licensed tea-room
Hidcote, Bartrim, Chipping
Campden
Tel: (038677) 703

HAMPSHIRE

The Vyne
Unlicensed tea-room
Sherborne St John, Basingstoke
Tel: (0256) 881337

HEREFORD & WORCESTER

Berrington Hall
Unlicensed tea-room
Leominster
Tel: (0568) 5721

Hanbury Hall
Unlicensed tea-room
Droitwich
Tel: (052784) 214

KENT

Chartwell
Licensed restaurant
Westerham
Tel: (0732) 866368

Sissinghurst Castle
Licensed tea-room
Sissinghurst, Cranbrook
Tel: (0580) 713097

LANCASHIRE

Rufford Old Hall
Unlicensed tea-room
Rufford, Nr Ormskirk
Tel: (0704) 821254

LINCOLNSHIRE

Belton House
Licensed restaurant
Nr Grantham
Tel: (0476) 66116

MERSEYSIDE

Speke Hall
Unlicensed tea-room
Liverpool
Tel: (051427) 7231

NORFOLK

Blickling Hall
Licensed restaurant
Blickling, Norwich
Tel: (0263) 733084

Felbrigg Hall
Licensed restaurant
Felbrigg, Norwich
Tel: (026375) 444

Oxburgh Hall
Unlicensed tea-room
Oxborough, King's Lynn
Tel: (36621) 258

NORTHANTS

Canons Ashby
Unlicensed tea-room
Daventry
Tel: (0327) 860044

NORTHERN IRELAND

The Argory (Co. Armagh)
Light refreshments
Moy, Dungannon, Co. Tyrone
Tel: (08687) 84753

Castle Ward
Unlicensed tea-room
Strangford, Downpatrick, Co.
Down
Tel: (039686) 204

Florence Court
Unlicensed tea-room
Nr Enniskillen, Co. Fermanagh
Tel: (036582) 249

Giant's Causeway
Unlicensed tea-room
Bushmills, Co. Antrim
Tel: (02657) 31582

Mount Stewart
Unlicensed tea-room
Newtownards, Co. Down
Tel: (024744) 387

NORTHUMBERLAND

Cragside
Licensed restaurant
Rothbury, Morpeth
Tel: (0669) 20134

Housesteads
Light refreshments
Bardon Mill, Hexham
Tel: (04984) 525

Wallington
Unlicensed restaurant
The Clock Tower Restaurant,
Wallington, Cambo, Morpeth
Tel: (067074) 274

NORTH YORKSHIRE

Beningbrough Hall
Licensed restaurant
Shipton-by-Beningbrough, York
Tel: (0904) 470715

Brimham Rocks
Unlicensed kiosk
Summerbridge, Nr Harrogate
Tel: (0423) 780688

Fountains Abbey & Studley Royal
Licensed restaurant
Studley Royal Park, Nr Ripon
Tel: (0765) 4246

Nunnington Hall
Unlicensed tea-room
Nunnington, York
Tel: (04395) 283

Treasurer's House
Licensed tea-room
Minster Yard, York
Tel: (0904) 646757

NOTTINGHAMSHIRE

Clumber Park
Unlicensed tea-room
Worksop
Tel: (0909) 484122

OXFORDSHIRE

Greys Court
Unlicensed tea-room
Rotherfield Greys,
Nr Henley-on-Thames
Tel: (04917) 529

SHROPSHIRE

Attingham Park
Unlicensed tea-room
Shrewsbury
Tel: (074377) 203

Carding Mill Valley
Unlicensed café
Chalet Pavilion, Church Stretton
Tel: (0694) 722631

Dudmaston
Unlicensed tea-room
Quatt, Bridgnorth
Tel: (0746) 780866

SOMERSET

Montacute House
Licensed café
Nr Yeovil
Tel: (0935) 824575

STAFFORDSHIRE

Moseley Old Hall
Unlicensed tea-room
Fordhouses, Wolverhampton
Tel: (0902) 782808

SUFFOLK

Flatford
Unlicensed café
Bridge Cottage, Flatford, East
Bergholt, Colchester
Tel: (0206) 298260

Ickworth
Licensed restaurant
Horringer, Bury St Edmunds
Tel: (028488) 270

Lavenham
Unlicensed tea-room
The Guildhall, Market Place,
Lavenham
Tel: (0787) 247646

SURREY

Box Hill
Licensed restaurant
Tadworth
Tel: (0306) 888793

Clandon Park
Licensed restaurant
West Clandon, Guildford
Tel: (0483) 222502

Claremont
Light refreshments
Portsmouth Road, Esher

Hatchlands
Unlicensed tea-room
East Clandon, Guildford
Tel: (0483) 222787

Polesden Lacey
Licensed restaurant
Nr Dorking
Tel: (0372) 56190

WALES

Chirk Castle
Licensed tea-room
Chirk, Clwyd
Tel: (0691) 777701

Erddig
Licensed tea-room
Wrexham, Clwyd
Tel: (0978) 355314

Penrhyn Castle
Licensed tea-room
Bangor, Gwynedd
Tel: (0248) 353084

Plas Newydd
Licensed tea-room
Llanfairpwll, Isle of Anglesey,
Gwynedd
Tel: (0248) 714795

Powis Castle
Licensed tea-room
Welshpool, Powys
Tel: (0938) 5499

WARWICKSHIRE

Baddesley Clinton
Licensed tea-room
Knowle, Solihull
Tel: (05643) 3294

Charlecote Park
Unlicensed tea-room
Wellesbourne, Warwick
Tel: (0789) 840277

Coughton Court
Unlicensed tea-room
Alcester
Tel: (0789) 762435

WEST SUSSEX

Nymans Garden
Light refreshments
Handcross, Nr Haywards Heath
Tel: (0444) 400002

Petworth House
Unlicensed tea-room
Petworth
Tel: (0798) 42207

Standen
Unlicensed tea-room
East Grinstead
Tel: (0342) 23029

WEST YORKSHIRE

East Riddlesden Hall
Unlicensed tea-room
Bradford Road, Keighley
Tel: (0535) 607075

WILTSHIRE

Stourhead
Licensed inn
The Spread Eagle Inn, Stourton, Nr
Warminster
Tel: (0747) 840587

Stourton Village Hall
Unlicensed tea-room
Stourton, Nr Warminster

Index

156

158